SASSY

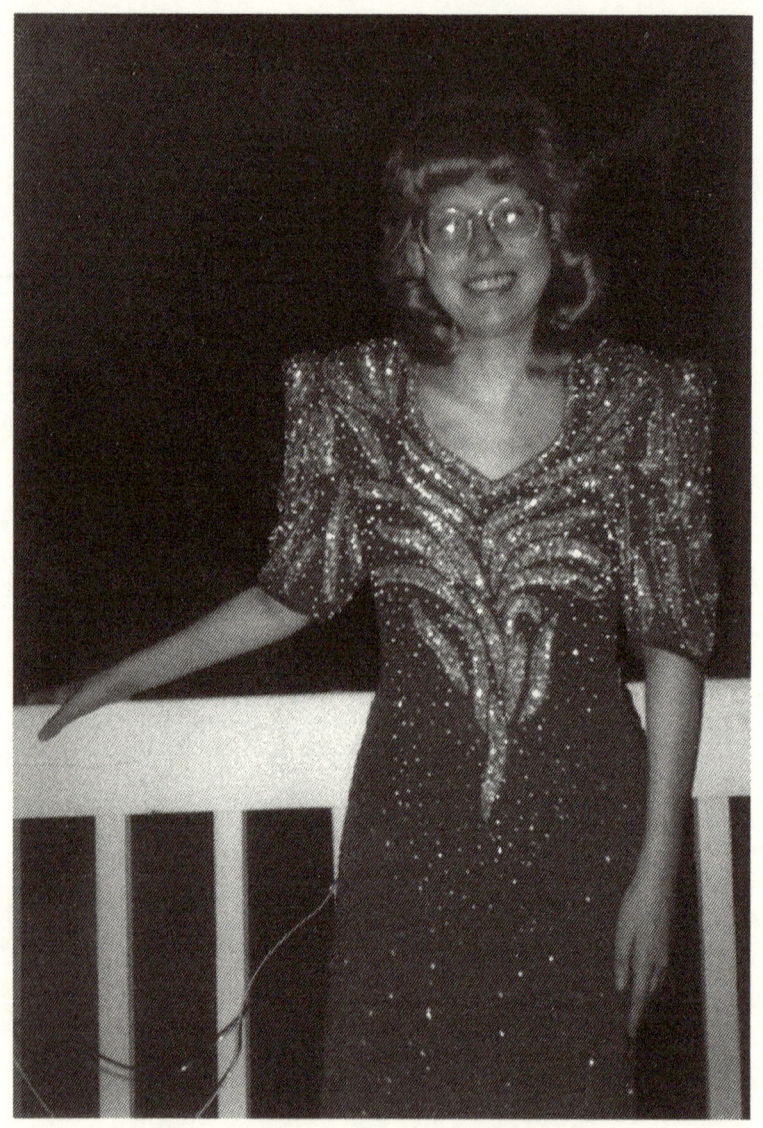

Vicky in the dress her angel purchased for her.

SASSY

THE FACE OF COURAGE

The story of Victoria Lynn Bowen's battle with Ewing's
Sarcoma Bone Cancer

THOMAS A. BOWEN

Writer's Showcase presented by *Writer's Digest*
San Jose New York Lincoln Shanghai

Sassy
The Face of Courage

Published by Writer's Showcase presented by *Writer's Digest*
an imprint of iUniverse.com, Inc.

For information address:
iUniverse.com, Inc.
620 North 48th Street
Suite 201
Lincoln, NE 68504-3467
www.iuniverse.com

Unless otherwise identified, Scripture quotations are from the King James
Version of the Bible.

ISBN: 0-595-00476-8

Printed in the United States of America

DEDICATION

This book is dedicated to two other families who battled Ewing's Sarcoma with Vicky. Kara Travis lost the battle with cancer shortly before Vicky did. Justin Terrell's cancer returned after his treatment was finished. The treatment of a bone marrow transplant took away his cancer for a second time. Justin lost his battle with cancer in 1999.

Vicky helped write the first part of this book, which takes you from "Why Me" to "Nurse Abuse." Vicky died before the book was finished. Her dad finished the book.

Doctor Kimo Stine, at Arkansas Children's Hospital taught those who were willing to learn about the effects of cancer. Many of the lessons I learned are recorded in the following paragraphs.

Cancers, which affect adults and children, are different. For every 100 adults diagnosed with cancer, only one child will be diagnosed with cancer. However, cancer is a major cause of death in children. In the past, the scope of cancer research focused on the major types of cancers, which affect the adult population. Only within the past ten to fifteen years has congress permitted research on children with childhood cancers. The amazing result is that children are starting to survive as a result of this resent research. Over 30 children's hospitals worldwide are linked together to find a cure for all the types of cancers which children can get. In Arkansas, it is Arkansas Children's Hospital that is working to find cures for cancer in children. Most of the kids over the age of 12 are treated in adult hospitals.

When a promising cancer agent (called chemotherapy) is discovered, it goes through laboratory testing to prove its ability to kill cancer cells, and not kill normal cells. The next step is to enter into a phase one study. In this phase, people with cancer are administered the chemotherapy for the sole purpose of finding out how much of the drug can be tolerated (therapeutic level) without causing unacceptable damage to normal tissue. The promise of curing the cancer is not guaranteed to any degree. Once the therapeutic level is established, and side effects are known, the drug enters phase two testing. Phase two testing determines the effectiveness of the chemotherapy on various types of tumors. When the chemotherapy is proven effective on a specific type of tumor, the Food and Drug Administration (FDA) then approves it as a cancer-fighting agent for that form of cancer. Today there are over 100 FDA approved chemotherapy drugs for the more than 50 types of cancer. It once took many years to move a drug to FDA approval. With new congressional legislation, drugs are moving to this level of approval much faster. It is important to remember that ten to fifteen years ago, children were not allowed, by law, to have access to phase one or phase two drugs. The chemotherapy that kills one form of cancer in an adult (and is FDA approved for that purpose) may not kill the same form of cancer in a child. Again, this is because cancer in children is different from cancer in adults.

In Arkansas, there will be 50 to 60 newly diagnosed cases of childhood cancer each year. By comparison, there will be 5,000 to 6,000 new adult cancer cases diagnosed in the state the same year. These become staggering numbers when you look at the nation as a whole. Leukemia and brain tumors are the most common forms of childhood cancers. Ewing's sarcoma is one of the most rare, with only 300 to 400 cases each year worldwide. Because of the small number of kids with Ewing's Sarcoma, it is important that all of the children's hospitals share their research information.

Ewing's sarcoma is now known to start in the nerve cells within the bones. It is during the period of adolescence growth that this form of cancer can occur. Once a Ewing's sarcoma cancer cell has formed, it rapidly multiplies. It takes over one billion cancer cells to produce a tumor large enough to be detected by present diagnostic studies, and within a few months the tumor can be large enough to cause death. Ewing's Sarcoma cells, like other cancer cells, desire to break off and locate in other parts of the body. It is like a dandelion that sends its seeds every where as the wind comes past. What is not understood is why one form of Ewing's sarcoma wants to find soft tissue, like the lungs and brain, while another form of Ewing's sarcoma wants to find other bones. The form of Ewing's sarcoma that seeks out other bones is the hardest to eradicate with today's FDA approved drugs.

Only recently has Arkansas Children's Hospital started participating in phase one testing on children. Insurance companies will have nothing to do with phase one studies. Grants and funding by the drug manufacturers are the primary sources of income for this type of study.

This book is written in honor to all of the people who are a part of cancer research for children.

CONTENTS

FOREWORD

Anyone affected by a significant emotional event will change his or her priorities in life overnight. Hobbies, social activities, leisure time, school, and work will all take on less importance as each day of your life passes. Deep down I knew this, but until Vicky was diagnosed with Ewing's sarcoma cancer it was only a superficial thought.

Every person has a place in his or her heart that hurts. For some this hurt is hidden away, but it is always there. It took a long time for me to allow that part of my heart to speak in the pages of this book. There are several places where the pain is still more than I can stand. For now the pages contain only part of the story. I am sure you will find where those places are. I ask that you will allow me the privilege to refrain from writing those stories right now.

I teach a boys group in our local church called "Royal Rangers." The boys are taught that there are four major areas you grow in. These are physically, mentally, spiritually, and socially. Each of these four areas is to be in balance to have a healthy life. When cancer came into my family, these areas tilted, and we had to regain control. By experience, I now know that these four areas are essential if individuals are going to survive the stresses of a significant emotional event like cancer and its treatments.

When you read through these pages about Vicky's struggle with cancer, you will see these areas tilt. And then you will see the balance return to her life through encounters with other people. If you allow your social life to collapse because of a significant emotional event like cancer, you will isolate yourself from the very sources that are necessary for survival.

It was important that I quickly climb the learning curve about cancer, treatment, and the emotional effects of this major illness. I had to learn how to interpret the results of blood tests. I reviewed each x-ray, CT scan, and MRI with the doctors.

The social workers and chaplains were the experts for learning about the emotional side of cancer. The book, *Everyone's Guide To Cancer Therapy,*[1] covers all types of cancer and chemotherapy with an overview of what cancer is. The American Cancer Society has a booklet on bone marrow transplants, which tells how blood is manufactured in the bones. The "Karing"[2] manual kept everything organized with places to record blood tests, hospital visits, and x-rays.

I always asked questions about every piece of information. The more I knew about what was happening, the better the doctors and nurses managed the treatments. Keeping a journal of my thoughts and feelings was very important.

I was ready at all times for a trip to the hospital or clinic. When platelets were low, red counts were low, or a fever set in, Vicky needed to go to the hospital or clinic quickly for treatment. I kept a change of clothes packed along with pajamas. I placed this suitcase where I could quickly grab it on the way to the hospital or clinic.

A tackle box made a perfect tool for storing medical supplies used every week at home. I kept this ready to take with me when Vicky went to the hospital or clinic.

I used the "Karing" manual to record medical history and I kept up with a calendar of treatments. I needed some type of system like this. I always took it with me to clinic visits and the hospital.

Most importantly, remember to take care of yourself. If you become a patient due to stress, someone will lose a primary advocate.

1 *Everyone's Guide to Cancer Therapy,* by Malin Dollinger, Somerville House Books Limited, ISBN 0-8362-2427-2

This book covers all types of cancer and all types of treatments in understandable terms.

2. Karing manual, by Charlotte Hawkins, 80601 Driver Rd., Wamic, OR 97063

Charlotte lost a child to cancer, and put this binder together to help other families organize the volumes of information about treatment. Cost is $25.00

ACKNOWLEDGEMENTS

Many people (who are a part of Vicky's story) should be mentioned. I will never know everyone who was involved since information about Vicky literally went around the world over the Internet and by word of mouth.

The doctors, nurses, and staff at Arkansas Children's Hospital, along with the county health nurses, provided the treatment and care that kept Vicky alive for nearly two years. Their inspiration and insight kept everyone's attitude as positive as possible. Vicky Davis with Arkansas Children's Dreams lifted Vicky's self esteem to the highest possible level.

Karen Wheaton is a special friend who ministered to Vicky and my family as no one else could. Karen continues to minister to us today. Carole, Sharon, Jenn, Laura, Ron, and Pat are special family friends. They are now family after Vicky adopted each one. Sharon allowed herself to become so close to Vicky that the two became real sisters.

Dade and Sheila Kindrix were our pastors who were always there. No matter what time of day, they were only a call away. Many times they were even closer.

The Johnson County Westside High School staff did so much to encourage Vicky. They made graduation and the prom special events. Vicky's classmates rallied to Vicky's side at every possible opportunity at home, school, and the hospital.

The staff and volunteers at Camp Barnabas helped Vicky transform from a girl into a young woman. Their inspiration and prayers literally pulled Vicky from the clutches of death more than once. A book about

Camp Barnabas was sent to a publisher in 1998. One of its chapters tells the story of Vicky and Sharon at camp in 1997.

Leta Miller, Burl Neal, and many other friends at work encouraged us and supported us in every possible way. Leta graciously donated to research a cure for Ewing's Sarcoma.

Sheila Martin was my English Composition teacher who showed me how to love writing. Without her as my mentor this book would not exist.

EDITORIAL METHOD

I asked Sheila Martin to edit the story of Vicky. She did so, and left me several questions to answer. Some of the questions were easy to answer, but the others were painful to address. The key question I had to answer was: "What do I see as the primary purpose of this book? Do I fall short in accomplishing these objectives?"

The primary purpose is to keep my promise to Vicky. I promised her that I would finish the story she started. So why did Vicky want to write a book? Vicky wanted all of the people who had any part in her struggle to know her story. There are those who prayed for her, those who provided various gifts to her, those who visited with her, and those who provided the medical care. Teens of today are flooded with the emotions of events like school shootings and car wrecks with the resultant death of their peers. Vicky believed that teens throughout the world wanted to know about such experiences with death. But, Vicky wanted to tell her peers about the silent killers like cancer. Vicky wanted all of her peers to know what it was like to die slowly. Most of all Vicky wanted these same peers to know that there was hope in the midst of sorrow.

The next objective did not exist until a few people were asked to read the unedited book. Individuals had no idea what it was like for kids to have cancer. No one really knew how a family struggles with a significant emotional event like cancer in a child. Vicky's many doctors encouraged me to publish the book. I met a young girl who lost both of her legs in a boating accident. She expressed the depression her doctors experienced when they did not know her outcome. This young girl learned that her doctors thought she died. But, she was alive and doing well. Vicky's story tells the complete human interface between the patient and the many medical professionals she encountered. My second objective then is to tell the world what it is like to lose a child to cancer as a parent, as a family, as a caregiver, and as a village. The world in general wants to know more about the youth of today. Vicky's story is a real look into the inner struggle kids face today. Cancer in and of itself is not the struggle. Simply searching to find a reason to face today is the struggle.

My final objective came out of Sheila Martin's observations. This objective also answered her question: "Why does the book stop so abruptly?" I was encouraged to be "brutally honest." I failed to tell the real story of the final hours of Vicky's life. I did so because I could not bear the pain of knowing that I failed in many areas. I had to admit my fears, anger, and blunders. Therefore the final objective is to tell the truth about the death of my daughter from my point of view.

Without writing this book, and asking for Sheila's comments, I would have run from the truth for years. I was in charge of writing the book. Therefore I felt in charge over cancer and death. But, death kept writing the last words. I had to struggle with death to finish the story. I trust that you will read the truth and realize that it is OK to fail when the pain of death swallows you. Without this knowledge those affected by death will continue to condemn themselves for what is normal. There is a huge difference between conviction and condemnation. Conviction will bring you to healing while condemnation will drive you to intense emotional pain. I experienced the painful truth of this first-hand. Sheila convicted me with her questions. I thank her very much for showing me that I can face the truth, and the truth set me free. Every reader must learn the truth about the grieving process. Healing is a life long process, and one never arrives. Some simply move along faster than others do. If we are not careful, you and I will find fault in others who are not as far along as we think they should be. Be careful in your comments to those who are in the process of grief recovery. A simple statement like "God is still able to help you" hurts those in the midst of grief. I would respond with the question: "When did He stop?"

My next question was to determine "Who is my targeted audience? Did I use the proper diction for the audience?" Since my audience does not normally use technical terms I had to change a lot of words. I was so used to the medical terms that I forgot that the reader would be lost. An example is a feed tube. How can I describe such a device in non-technical terms? The best description is that it looks like a piece of spaghetti three feet long. Its stiffness is between that of cooked and uncooked spaghetti. Using a feed tube is like trying to put this half-cooked noodle down your nose. The major difference is that the tube is made of rubber and you can't eat it or bite it in half.

The next question dealt with format. Sheila observed that "this book is a sort of diary that is not extremely organized." Then she asked, "Is this the format you want?" I did not know what the best format was for the book. I never wrote a book before. I started with daily journal entries as a skeleton for the book. I then went back to hang words on the skeleton just like adding muscle. I then went back once again and added what I considered to be the finishing touches much like covering a body with skin. Sheila's observation made me take another look. What I left out was the heart, brain and lungs. I needed to give life to the story. The story was stiff like a robot. I went back and added life to the pages. Yet there are still places that are stiff like a robot. This is done on purpose to reflect the way I was living at the time. I simply took one step at a time doing the analytical work of a busy dad. Again this is an area where I failed to see that I was doing things to stay busy without taking time to enjoy life. Doctor Stine kept trying to tell me to take one day at a time and enjoy it. I thought I was doing better than that by trying to fit cancer into a schedule. Cancer seemed to have a way of messing up my schedule every now and then.

The last question was: "Do you want the reader to get an accurate picture of the struggles your entire family went through?" Sheila noticed that my wife, Vanessa, seemed to get lost in the story. In reality she did. I forgot to take care of my family and myself while Vicky struggled with cancer. I was asked to write even more "straight from the heart" about the many ranges of emotions my family experienced. Again Sheila pointed out an area I failed in. Vicky's social worker told me one day that half of all married couples who have a child with cancer file for divorce. I realize now how close Vanessa and I came to this same encounter. I hope that every reader will catch hold of this major point. Families cannot be neglected when a child has cancer. The family will need major care for many years. I know that this is more than most families, churches, and communities can bear. This is why Vanessa and I started a foundation for kids with cancer and other life threatening issues. Through the efforts of this foundation Vanessa and I want to bring hope to many of the families in and around Arkansas whose children struggle with life and death every day.

Thank you Sheila for editing Vicky's book. It is now my task to get Vicky's story into the hands of the intended audience. God puts people in our paths at just the right time, doesn't He?

Sincerely,

Thomas

WHY ME?

A t the young age of 6, Victoria Lynn Bowen (Vicky) was diagnosed with complex partial seizures. The epilepsy causes a blank stare, generates a repetitive motion, and short-term memory is lost during the time of the seizure. Through many years and tests, Victoria found out that stress and sequential operations, such as schoolwork trigger the seizures. The seizures are controlled by medication, unless there is stress with sequencing. At the age of 15, Victoria started questioning "why me?" Victoria's struggle with epilepsy would prove to be insignificant compared to the battle ahead of her.

Four months before Thanksgiving of 1995, Victoria fell out of her bed onto her left shoulder. The shoulder was x-rayed, and no damage was found. Victoria wore a sling for a few weeks, and her arm healed. Two weeks before Thanksgiving, I noticed Victoria having difficulty with her left arm again. She put the sling back on since Victoria remembered bumping her shoulder. As Thanksgiving approached, Victoria's left arm got worse. On November 24 and 25, 1995, Victoria attended the Youth Convention in Little Rock with her church youth group. At the convention she needed help getting dressed. Victoria's left arm simply would not lift up high enough to go into her dresses. The youth pastors pointed this out, and Vanessa (Mom) and I made an appointment with the family pediatrician in Russellville. Victoria's left arm had the symptoms of a dislocated shoulder, but the x-ray showed a much different story. Situated over the left shoulder blade between the ribs and arm was a soft tissue mass. An orthopedic surgeon, Doctor Nicholas, at the University of Arkansas for Medical Sciences (UAMS), in Little Rock was contacted. He requested two additional tests—a MRI of the shoulder and a bone scan.

We met with Doctor Nicholas at the end of the week, and reviewed all the results including the x-ray from four months earlier. Doctor Nicholas was very sure that Victoria had cancer. Specifically, he was confident that this was a rare form of bone cancer called "Ewing's sarcoma." Victoria was scheduled for further tests at Children's Hospital. The additional tests showed the tumor to be wrapped around the nerves for the left arm along with the arm's blood supply and lymph drain. Victoria was scheduled to enter Children's Hospital for a biopsy.

The three days at Children's Hospital in Little Rock, Arkansas were filled with tests and meetings. The scans revealed that the cancer was in the left and right hipbones, the left leg bone above the knee, and the left shoulder blade. As a result of the test results, bone marrow was removed from both hips to test for leukemia. Victoria was put to sleep for this test. Nothing was found in the bone marrow.

The soft tumor in the left shoulder was growing out of the shoulder blade, and was limiting arm motion. We met with the oncology group during the week, and came to know Doctor Kimo Stine and his nurse Carol Godfrey. A dual intravenous line, known as a port, was installed in the right side. The central line entered above the collarbone, went into the blood vessel, and stopped at the heart. A few stitches held it in place. Now there was the wait. Doctor Nicholas performed the biopsy, and he was 100% sure that Victoria had Ewing's sarcoma. The pathologist's report was needed to make it official. Victoria was asking once again, "why me?" Vanessa and I were praying for a non-cancerous pathology report.

Emotions were flooding our lives. I couldn't believe that cancer was really there. Vanessa was in a state of denial. Vanessa believed that the cancer would just go away, or that the pathologist's report would reveal a simple infection. Victoria was scheduled to return to Children's

Hospital on Wednesday to start chemotherapy. Vanessa and I had to be trained in the care of the port before going home.

Victoria insisted on going to church Sunday morning. She wanted to tell the church "thank you for praying for me." Victoria also wrote a letter to the editor of the Graphic Newspaper stating her appreciation to the community for holding her up through the upcoming months of chemotherapy.

A special chair was set up for Victoria in the teen Sunday school class. I was worried about the pain in her left shoulder, but she did fine. Following Sunday school, the chair was brought upstairs. I set a drink of water by Victoria, and then joined the choir. From the choir loft I saw Victoria trying to reach the water. She was in great pain, and could not reach the glass. I left the choir and joined Victoria. She wanted a drink and a pain pill.

Prior to Pastor Dade Kindrix preaching, Victoria was invited to the front of the church to address the congregation. Victoria had asked the pastor for an opportunity to talk with the church. Victoria was in pain, but she sat and spoke as I held the microphone for her. Victoria told the church that she made it through the surgery for the biopsy. And, just like this surgery, she was going to make it through the chemotherapy. I took the microphone and explained that Victoria enjoyed Karen Wheaton's music. Victoria was holding onto the song about a miracle coming down the dusty road. Our son then played the song for the church while Victoria hugged me. I couldn't hold back the tears. Following the song I took Victoria back to her seat.

We set out to return to Children's Hospital on Wednesday. Our two-year-old daughter was left with the Dove family at church. Our two sons stayed at home with their cousin Shawnee. When we arrived at the hospital, the pathologist report was not in. What an emotional day, and weekend, that followed. The mass in Victoria's shoulder was now the size of a tennis ball pushing out of the shoulder. I began to wonder if the cancer would grow out of the skin.

We were sent home with instructions to check in each day for the pathologist report. On the way home we stopped at the American Cancer Society. Vanessa picked up three videotapes. One was called "Hair Balls on My Pillow." The other two dealt with the side effects of chemotherapy. Victoria picked out a wig in preparation for her hair to fall out. The wig was a little lighter than her normal brown color. It was a longer style, and it really looked good on her. Her hair had more curls than the new wig.

On Friday we were instructed to come to Children's Hospital on Monday at 11:00 a.m. On Monday, December 18, the pathologist's report was in, and Victoria did have Ewing's sarcoma. She was started on her first round of chemotherapy. The many different types of cancer and the different types of chemotherapy drugs overwhelmed us. The cancer was growing fast, and was doubling in size every 14 to 28 days. A new drug called "topotecan" had great potential for this type of cancer. Morphine was administered to control the pain in the shoulder. Victoria, her sister, Vanessa, and I stayed at a motel in Little Rock. The drug was administered for 4 hours each day on an outpatient basis. Since topotecan was not FDA approved for Ewing's sarcoma, the insurance company did not pay any of this treatment. Applications for Medicaid and Medicare were submitted.

On the first night of chemotherapy Victoria was doing all right. The medication given to prevent nausea made her very tired.

On the second day, Victoria's electrolytes were off. She did not drink enough water through the night to flush the chemotherapy out of the blood. Victoria was given extra fluids by IV on day two. Vanessa and I made sure that Victoria drank a lot of fluids. On Tuesday evening Victoria asked to go to Chuck E. Cheese Pizza for dinner. Victoria met the night manager who was a survivor of cancer and chemotherapy. The two exchanged phone numbers.

On Wednesday Victoria's electrolyte level was normal—she drank enough. The chemotherapy was really starting to drain Victoria's energy. Wednesday night Victoria was not able to walk to dinner. She experienced severe nausea and stomach cramps. She called her new friend from Chuck E. Cheese just to talk about her feelings. Thursday and Friday continued to drain her energy.

Following treatment Thursday, Vanessa wanted to go shopping at Michael's for craft supplies. Victoria had to sit in a chair because she was too tired to go on. I had to take her to the bathroom because of nausea. Victoria could barely hold herself up to walk. I was very irritated knowing that the insurance would not pay to place Victoria in the hospital. Thursday night Victoria had to call Sister Sheila to talk. Victoria was really feeling down, and asking "why me?"

We went home Friday with a trunk full of medical supplies, and home health scheduled to come to our house twice a week. On Sunday Victoria was feeling much better, and again wanted to go to church. Victoria shared her experiences with her youth group.

Monday through Friday of the first week at home was filled with home health visits, intravenous line flushes and dressing changes, lab work, and injections to increase the white blood cell production. Not only does chemotherapy kill cancer cells it also kills fast growing cells like blood, hair, and the lining of the mouth.

We had Victoria home for Christmas. She did well physically for having gone through chemotherapy. But, emotionally Victoria was devastated. She found comfort in talking with Sister Sheila and her teen-age daughter, Marcie. We watched her blood counts for the next two weeks. We watched for a fever or signs of an infection. We read all of the literature we could find about Ewing's sarcoma. We thought we were ready for everything.

Monday of the second week at home was Victoria's best day. She was feeling so good that she took her sling off of her arm. She went to visit her friend Amanda for a few hours. On Tuesday, Victoria's arm started to hurt again. We attributed it to not wearing her sling the day before.

From the time Victoria went home on December 22 until January 3, the tumor continued to visibly shrink each day. But, from the 4th to 8th, it started to grow again. Victoria's left arm swelled, giving her great pain. Morphine was needed to tolerate the pain. Victoria did not attend church Sunday, January 7. Sunday afternoon we left for a motel in Little Rock. Victoria's shoulder was swelling much faster on Sunday than any other day. During the night I had to give Victoria morphine several times to control the pain.

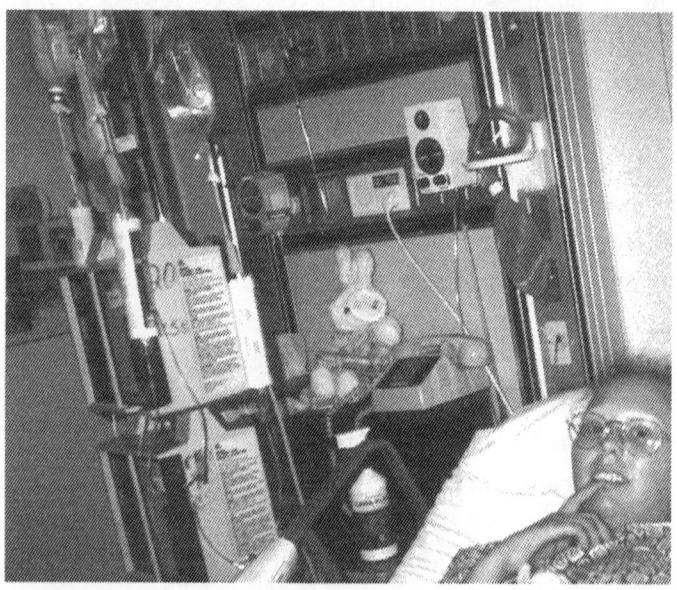

Vicky back in her room after the first stay in intensive care.

CANCER IS A FAMILY AFFAIR

On Monday morning, January 8, we arrived at the clinic at 9:00 a.m. Doctor Stine did not want to use a second round of topotecan because the tumor grew back so quickly. Victoria was admitted to Children's Hospital for chemotherapy drugs called iphosfamide and VP-16. Since these were FDA approved drugs, the insurance company allowed Victoria to be admitted to the hospital. These stronger forms of FDA approved chemotherapy were used for the next five days.

The side effects of VP 16 are low blood counts, nerve numbness and tingling, shortness of breath, rapid heart rate, loss of hair, loss of appetite, altered taste and smell, nausea, vomiting, sore mouth, diarrhea, and loss of fluids and electrolytes. The side effects of iphosfamide are bladder bleeding and inflammation, kidney malfunction, low blood counts, sleepiness and confusion, hair loss, liver malfunction, water overload, lung scarring, nausea, and vomiting.

The side effects were very traumatic for Victoria. There were the mouth sores, sore throat, nausea, and loss of appetite. Victoria's pain in the shoulder was so intense that the Children's Hospital pain team set up a morphine pump to give morphine continuously.

At 11:30 on Monday morning, Victoria went to x-ray for a CT scan of her shoulder. Victoria could barely lay still because of the intense pain in the left shoulder. Victoria went to the third floor, Gold section, and room 3141. The first round of chemotherapy was started at 6:00 p.m.

On Wednesday Victoria started having trouble keeping her pills down because of nausea. Her appetite went away, and her fluid intake dropped off.

On Friday Victoria started to run a fever. Her throat was so raw that she could no longer swallow her medications without choking on them. Her temperature was 102. From Friday, January 12, until Wednesday, January 17, the fever persisted despite antibiotics and Tylenol. Victoria's infection fighting white blood count dropped to zero as the chemotherapy attacked the fast growing cells. A yeast infection in her mouth quickly moved into her lungs. Oxygen levels in the blood dropped from a normal of 100 percent to 40 percent.

Vanessa and I went home Tuesday after being at the hospital for a week, and planned to return the following evening. Shannon and Marcie were going to visit Victoria both days.

Marcie was visiting with Victoria Wednesday evening when she was transferred to intensive care where she was placed on life support. Her temperature was 106. Vanessa and I returned from home just after she was transferred to the Pediatric Intensive Care Unit (PICU). Victoria needed a lot of blood. Whole blood is separated into three products, which includes red blood cells, platelets, and plasma. I learned that white blood cells cannot be transfused. The body must make its own white blood cells. There was a special injection that helped the bone marrow speed up the production of white blood cells. Machines were breathing for her, medications were controlling blood pressure, and two cooling blankets were required to control temperature. Victoria was given a 40 percent chance to survive the night. Victoria's lungs, kidneys, and liver were damaged by the infection. Wednesday evening services were in progress at our church when I called the pastor. Brother Dade and Sister Sheila left for the hospital the moment services were closed.

Prayer meetings were organized where the church family could pray specifically for Victoria and our family. I realized that I could not heal my daughter by myself. I had to place Victoria into the hands of God, and reach her through God's nature of prayer. Romans 5:3 and 4 states: "knowing that tribulation worketh patience; and patience, experience; and experience, hope." I had to learn to be patient in prayer through this time of tribulation.

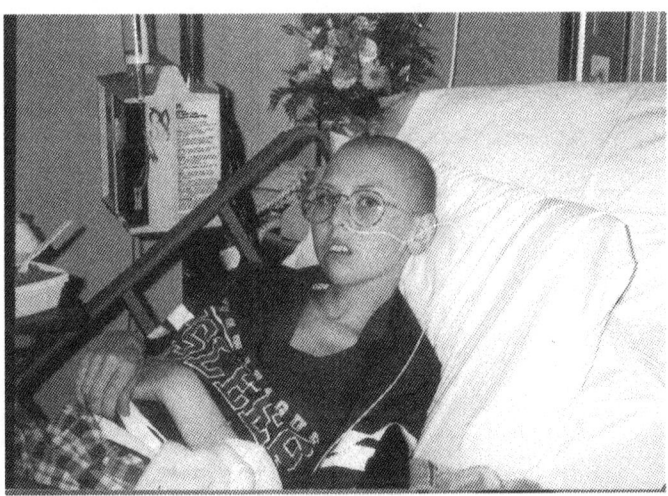

Vicky wanted to eat. The feed tube could be removed if
Vicky ate the spaghetti on the table.

Intensive Care

Victoria's lungs had the appearance of pneumonia on the x-rays. The lungs were flushed and sampled. The results of the lung sample showed a fungus growing. Antibiotics for the specific fungus were started. Victoria's blood pressure stabilized, and her color was much better.

We requested a letter from Dr. Stine describing Victoria's condition and chemotherapy schedule to deliver to Dial-A-Page. The manager at Dial-A-Page provided us with a pager. Vanessa felt much better knowing she could reach me immediately.

Terry Nichols, one of the church deacons, visited with Vanessa and I for several hours. His presence, compassion, and prayers were a great strength for us. Many other friends from church, work, and the hospital came to visit.

On Thursday, January 18, Vanessa and I checked into a local motel to get some much-needed rest. I called PICU every four hours to check on Victoria's status. We were glad that the pager never went off.

Our son, Terry, experienced vehicle troubles at home. Charlie and Johnna Boone drove me home on Friday to help Terry. I returned to the hospital on Saturday with Brother Dade and Sister Sheila. Along the way, they picked up their son and his wife, Marcus and Abby. The many visitors comforted Vanessa and me.

Each morning, I would meet with the PICU doctors, and discuss all test results. I soon learned what each value on the blood tests meant, and which medications were used for correction. The PICU staff welcomed taking an interest at this level, and it helped me feel involved in

Victoria's case. I wrote everything down that I learned. I read books at the hospital library to gain more knowledge. It was something I could do. Vanessa spent hours crafting blankets out of yarn. The two of us spent little time together.

On January 22, the ventilator oxygen setting was reduced from 50 percent to 40 percent. The lower setting meant that Victoria's lungs were getting better. Victoria's platelet level was low, and she was given one unit of platelets and a unit of fresh frozen plasma. Victoria looked real puffy, and her chin and chest touched because of fluids leaking out of the blood vessels. She had already gained twenty pounds of fluid weight.

Victoria's white blood count started increasing on the 23rd. On the 24th, Victoria become more alert. She could blink her eyes, and move her fingers. I went to work for the first time since Victoria was placed in PICU. Vanessa and I were asked not to talk or touch Victoria in any manner that would startle her. Vanessa and I wanted to see Victoria's reactions. But, we didn't want to have any troubles, and we complied with the doctor's request.

Debbie Cole was one of my co-workers. She volunteered to keep our youngest daughter, Stacy, for as long as necessary. Debbie also made arrangements for Stacy to attend Shinn's day care with Debbie's daughter. Brady and Aleah Duff were members of our church. The Duff family volunteered to take our youngest son, Windle, on the weekends for as long as necessary. There were many other friends who helped with other responsibilities at home and at work. We left our 18-year-old son, Terry, in charge of our home in Johnson County.

Vanessa and I moved into the Ronald McDonald House next to the hospital on January 25 after living eight days in the PICU waiting room. The PICU waiting room has a unique culture where everyone has a common bond: a suffering child. We were welcomed by this special family, and given a tour of the basics. The showers, laundry room, location of linens, storage area, and sleeping arrangements are important to everyone. You are soon a part of this culture, and take up the role of showing newcomers to the room.

The Ronald McDonald house was just like a home. Sally was the director, and she became like a mom to us. Each employee had chores to do as did the occupants of each room. Our responsibility was to vacuum the upstairs hallways each day. Each bedroom has its own sink, and two beds. There is a men and women's common shower on each floor, and a large family room downstairs. There is an indoor and outdoor play area for the children. There are several kitchens in the house with donated foods for the occupants to prepare. On special occasions various groups provide a lovely meal for the entire house. On one occasion, one of the local airlines celebrated their anniversary with the McDonald's House family. Until you are in a situation like PICU, you don't know that this kind of love abounds.

Dr. Kimo Stine asked Sandra Still to visit with us. Sandra's son had Ewing's sarcoma in his hip four years ago. Sandra encouraged us with her personal testimony.

Several times Victoria was allowed to wake up by suspending the sedating medications. Each time she would start fighting the ventilator, and set off the peak pressure alarm. If the peak pressure goes too high, the lungs could rupture and collapse. The sedating medications would be turned back on.

The Beta Club from Victoria's school was in town on January 26 and 27. On Saturday, January 27, Mrs. Bean, Christie Grigsby, Amanda Marrow, and our son Terry came to visit Victoria. Amanda obtained permission to have pictures taken of her and Victoria in PICU.

From January 17 until February 18, Victoria lived in intensive care at Children's Hospital. She was on the ventilator until February 14th. On Tuesday, February 6, Vanessa and I consulted with the oncology department about Victoria's next round of chemotherapy. We were now one week late with the chemotherapy schedule. The tumor site in the left arm did not show any signs of growth. But, how long before the tumor would start growing again? On Wednesday, February 7, the doctors from all departments involved in Victoria's care met for a team meeting. At the meeting we discussed the health of her lungs, the response to the last round of chemotherapy, the need for the next round of chemotherapy, and all potential complications. None of the literature we studied covered any of this. I kept a journal, and recorded all of my emotions as the hours turned into days and the days into weeks.

In the Bible, James states that if anyone lacks wisdom let him or her ask for it from the Lord. Vanessa and I prayed going into this meeting. Without chemotherapy it would take one to two weeks for Victoria's lungs to heal enough to come off the ventilator. Then there was the time of recovery and weaning off of the many narcotics. The real goal of Victoria's illness was to cure the cancer. To wait placed that goal out of reach.

The doctors, Vanessa, and I agreed that adriamycin and vincristine chemotherapy should be given right away. These were two additional FDA approved chemotherapy treatments. There were special complications simply because Victoria was in intensive care. This was a place where very sick kids were, and the last thing Victoria needed when the chemotherapy dropped her white blood count was an infection. To protect her, Victoria was placed into isolation and no visitors were allowed. The side effects of adriamycin are hair loss, anemia, low blood counts, red coloration of urine, cardiac toxicity, skin cracking, nausea, vomiting, sore mouth, diarrhea, iron loss, and loss of appetite. The side effects of vincristine are numbness, tingling fingers and feet, hair loss, loss of nerve function (foot drop and partial paralysis), low blood counts, nausea, vomiting, constipation, sore mouth and throat, difficulty chewing or swallowing, dry mouth, altered taste and smell, and increased uric acid. Victoria did well with the chemotherapy.

On February 12, Brian Patrick Hargiss came to visit Victoria. He heard about Victoria's struggles, and felt impressed to sing to her. Brian took out his guitar and started singing to Victoria in PICU. The whole floor turned quiet as the healing words of praise were sung.

"The angels of God are singing with you in Victory. You are one with Him, and thy name is Victory! Victoria. May God bless you and keep you in the cleft of his hand."

Brian Patrick Hargiss

Victoria was removed from the ventilator on February 13 with success, but her right vocal cord was paralyzed from the trauma of the tube in her throat. In order to leave intensive care, Vicky had to have 24 hours without a fever. From Thursday to Saturday, she ran a fever. Finally, on February 18, Vicky was released from intensive care. Now Victoria required physical and occupational therapy to relearn the tasks of eating, walking, and talking. This would take a long time. The lining of her eyes dried out, and the cornea started to break down. The medications to correct the eyes were very painful. Just the smell of food made Victoria violently sick. Nourishment came in the form of intravenous (IV) bags.

Victoria wanted to be called Vicky by all of the therapists. There was respiratory, speech, physical, and occupational therapy. Vicky had a special beanbag that looked like a cow. She would tease Mike, the physical therapist, by throwing it at him. As this game continued, Vicky's arm gained strength.

At first Vicky was strapped in a wheel chair. Slowly she gained strength through exercises. After several weeks of therapy, Vicky was able to walk 50 feet with a walker. Another round of VP-16 and iphosfamide chemotherapy was administered. Vicky went into a chemical coma as toxic levels in her body increased when the kidneys broke down the chemotherapy drugs. She came out of the coma the following day once chemotherapy was stopped after four of the scheduled five days. The fifth day of chemotherapy was cancelled.

"We are praying for you at school."

Mrs. Bean

"I am believing God for your complete healing! Even better than before."
                                                    Stella Crawford

"I was in last weekend, and praying for you. Today you look great! See what prayer can do."

                                    Rita Odom, RN Nursing Supervisor

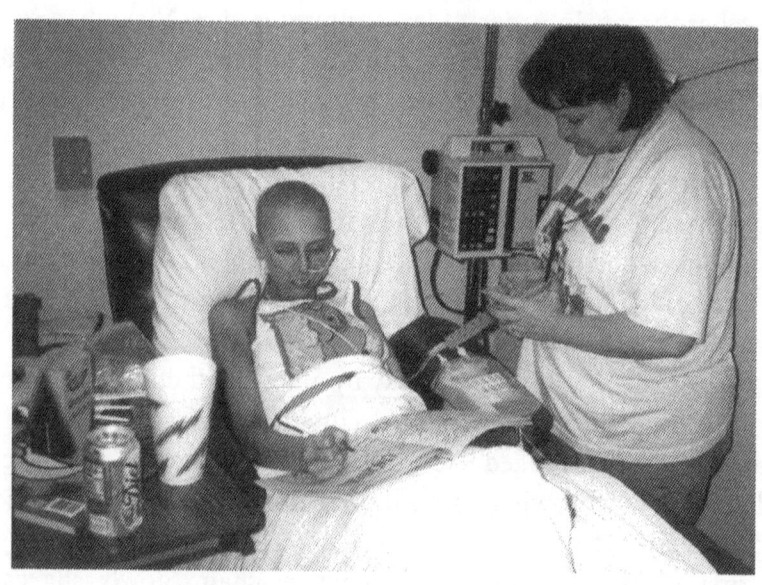

Vicky was receiving a unit of platelets.

THE NEED FOR MOTIVATION

At first, Vicky was bothered by the loss of her hair. One afternoon, she asked her nurse, Rhonda, to get the wig out of the closet. Knowing that Vicky needed to be cheered up, Rhonda put the wig on herself, and left the room. Rhonda recruited the help of other nurses on the 3-Gold ward. Rhonda added inches to her bust size, and returned to Vicky's room with an audiotape. Rhonda, and all of the nurses, sang "Turn Your Radio On," and danced before Vicky. It worked; Vicky came alive. She accused Rhonda of looking like Dolly. The more Vicky tried to retrieve her wig, the louder the group sang. "Turn Your Radio On" became the theme song of the day in Vicky's room, and each day Vicky cheered up more and more.

Brian Patrick Hargiss returned to the hospital to sing for Vicky now that she was out of intensive care. Brian asked Vicky if she remembered him singing to her in intensive care. She did not remember him being there, but she listened to the tape he left. Brian sang to Vicky for nearly two hours.

Victoria went into Children's Hospital on January 8, and came home on March 27. On the day of discharge, she dressed up in a new outfit, and put on her wig. On the way to the elevator, there was a round of applause from all of the nursing staff and doctors on the 3-Gold floor. The first place Vicky wanted to stop at was Wal-Mart. Part of the equipment to take home was two IV pumps. One was for fluids and vitamins, and the other was for fats and proteins. Both pumps were required 12 hours each night. Vanessa and I had to be trained in the use of the pumps before we could go home.

On Friday, March 29, Vicky met the Christian artist, Karen Wheaton, in Fort Smith. It was a wonderful evening put together by the TLC Foundation. The TLC Foundation is a Christian foundation seeking to lift the spirits of kids with serious illnesses. Vicky started the evening with a makeup makeover at Dillard's. She then went to the convention center where Karen's road manager presented Vicky with a dozen red roses. The vice president of the TLC foundation presented Vicky with another dozen roses. During the concert, Karen addressed Vicky and sang her favorite song about a miracle coming down a dusty road. Following the concert Vicky went back stage to meet Karen. Karen presented Vicky a special gift, CD's, and T-shirts. The evening came to an end at Western Sizzlin where Vicky ate her favorite foods: okra pickles, olives, grated cheese, and gummy bears. At the midnight hour, the TLC foundation presented Vicky with a jogging suit in full belief that Vicky would be out of her wheel chair, and jogging again very soon. Vicky and Karen wrote frequently. Vicky called Karen every now and then especially when the "why me?" question came up.

As expected with chemotherapy, Vicky's blood counts dropped through the week. On April 1 she came down with an infection when her immune system went away. Vicky was rushed back to Children's Hospital where she stayed until April 8. She was given antibiotics, and a growth factor to increase the white blood count. On April 5, the results of cultures identified the presence of a rare infection in her IV port, and the port was removed. Vicky experienced a slight sting when the port tubing was pulled out of her vein.

Vicky went home and stayed until her next round of chemotherapy on April 15. She continued to grow stronger by exercising. A physical therapist came to the house twice a week to work with Vicky. She could walk from one end of the house to the other, and could fix her own snacks without assistance. She went to church, Wal-Mart, and out to eat for more cheese and gummy bears.

Vicky was admitted to Children's Hospital on April 15 for a new IV port and chemotherapy. The three days of chemotherapy started on April 15 went well, and Vicky went home on April 18. Her blood count dropped as the chemotherapy did its work, and Vicky required 3 units of red blood on the 23rd. On the 25th, Vicky ran a fever again, and she was rushed to the emergency room at Children's Hospital. Her fluid inventory and platelet level was very low. Blood cultures revealed a fast growing strepp infection of the blood. On Friday Vicky's blood pressure and oxygen level dropped, and she was rushed to intensive care. A catheter was inserted in her groin. Vanessa and I moved into the Ronald McDonald house again as soon as there was an opening. This time our chores were cleaning of the tables in the dining area. Vanessa and I took turns visiting with Vicky. Vanessa used the quiet time to work on crafts.

Vicky spent the next three days receiving blood products, blood pressure medication, and antibiotics. She was released from intensive care on Monday. The doctors in PICU could administer larger doses of medications than could the doctors on the wards. These larger doses turned Vicky's condition around.

Vicky continued to need antibiotics to fight the infection. She was given a growth factor each day to increase bone marrow white blood cell production. The infection was cleared up, and Vicky was given four more units of red blood just in time to go on a "dream trip" sponsored by Arkansas Children's Dreams.

Ken Abbot, with Arkansas Children's Dreams, met us for dinner the night before the dream started. Vicky did not like the first restaurant because they did not have spaghetti. Vicky wanted to go to Pizza Hut, but they were closed for repairs. Ken led the way to the Macaroni Grill for spaghetti. Vicky would not eat anything that evening, and she did not want to talk to anyone. The spaghetti at the Macaroni Grill was excellent, but Vicky did not have an appetite. Everyone was concerned that Vicky might not tolerate the dream vacation.

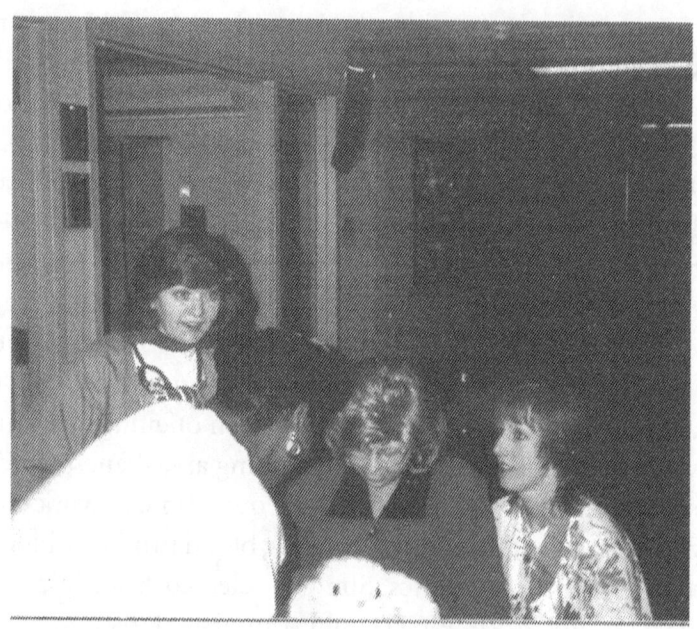

Vicky receiving instructions from her nurses.

A Child's Dream

Vicki Davis, the director of Arkansas Children's Dreams, arranged to send Vicky to Disneyland in California. Vanessa, Vicky, Windle, and I spent 5 days in California. One family at Children's Hospital who recently returned from there stated, "You won't want to come back to the reality of cancer and chemotherapy." Vicky had a wonderful time at Disneyland once she realized there were lots of stores to shop at. The flight to California according to Vicky was long and boring. Her brother, Windle, saw things completely different, and was excited the whole flight. Wheel chairs were waiting on Vicky at all of the airports. When we arrived at the Disney motel, Vicky wanted to go to bed, but we made her get out. Once she saw the store in the bottom of the motel, the vacation started. Vicky shopped until I dropped.

Dinner at Micky's dinner was special. We celebrated Windle's birthday, and Vicky laughed with all of the characters. The following day in the park was a race from one store to another. Vicky bought T-shirts, key rings, an umbrella, and lots of candy. We ate lunch at the Mexican restaurant in the park, and Vicky ate her enchilada, beans, and dip. She also drank as she was instructed. Dinner was at the Monorail Cafe where Vicky ate most of her spaghetti.

On the way to Universal Studios we stopped to see my sister (Vicky's aunt). Vicky climbed up the stairs to the apartment stating that it was no problem for a "Sassy" girl. Vicky's aunt gave us three containers of dip and four bags of chips for Vicky to snack on.

At Universal Studios Vicky and Windle enjoyed the tram ride on the back lot. Windle sat in the front right seat, and saw King Kong face to face. Vicky liked the earthquake the most. We ended the evening on the shopping strip where Vicky tried on hats with hair sewn in them. The leather hat with streaked hair brought the greatest laughs. We ate dinner in a country and western restaurant where Vicky watched the cowboys more than her dinner.

The last day we went to visit family and the beach. Vicky and Windle visited with their grandpa, grandma, several aunts, and lots of cousins. Grandpa gave Vicky money to go shopping with. We walked along the boardwalk of Ventura beach with the wind in our face and the smell of salty air. There was a pleasant peace as we watched the birds and waves dance as the sun set. We ate dinner in a Mexican restaurant that Vanessa and I ate in years ago called Sal's. Vicky ate all of her enchilada, all of her beans, and half of the avocado dip. We then went to a factory outlet mall, and shopped until it closed.

I drove back to the motel at Universal Studios and put Vicky in the spa. Vicky enjoyed being able to move her feet and legs freely. On the way back into the motel, Vicky started to cry. When I asked her what was wrong, she stated that she could no longer feel any pain in her legs. I could not hold back the tears of joy. For the remainder of the trip Vicky set aside her walker and wheel chair, and walked on her own. This was indeed a wonderful dream.

Vicky enjoyed the flight home. She was able to board both planes on her own. She drank the cokes and ate the peanuts. Back in Little Rock Vicky wanted a hamburger and onion rings at Shoneys. Vicky finished half of the onion rings, and most of the hamburger.

On the way back to Children's Hospital the next morning, Vicky phoned the nurses at the hospital. Vicky told the nurse, Janet, that she was still in California, and was not coming back. Vicky told Janet about the gifts she bought for Janet and Rhonda while at Disneyland, but she was going to keep them for herself. Vicky enjoyed being "Sassy."

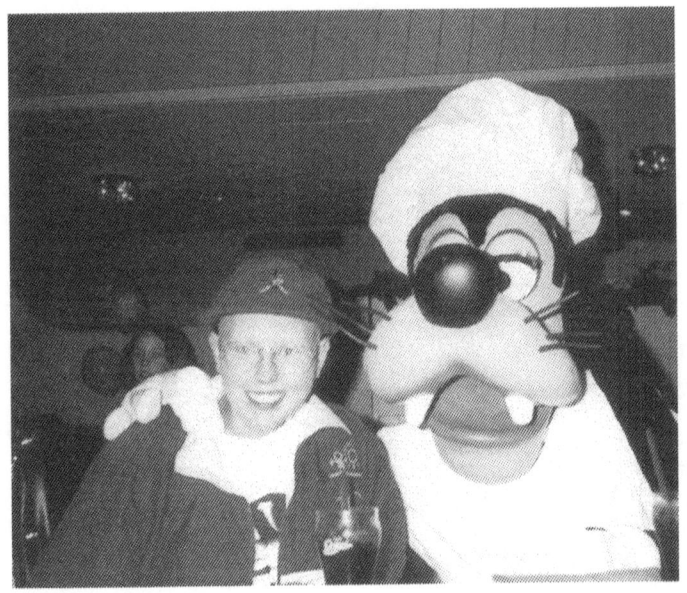

Vicky eating dinner with Goofy at Disneyland.

NICKNAMES

Vicky was placed back in the hospital May 13th for the next round of VP-16 and iphosfamide chemotherapy. Vicky was "Sassy" to the core with the nurses. It was more than a game Vicky played with her nurses. There was a friendship growing between the nurses and this young girl devastated by cancer.

To help with the toxic side effects of chemotherapy experienced last time; Vicky was given a drug called methalene blue. It stings like turpentine, and looks like India ink, and Vicky nicknamed it "love potion number 9." Thursday night through Saturday Vicky became very disoriented and weak. These symptoms were still there, but to a lesser degree Sunday night. Vicky's love potion was working. Vicky's white blood count dropped, and she ran a fever through the night. Vicky was able to walk to the sink and brush her teeth. Vicky showed the video of her dream vacation to the nurses Rhonda and Janet. Vicky and the nurses teased each other over many of the events captured on video. Janet stated that Vicky was getting bossy, but not quite sassy. Vicky tried to rise above bossy to sassy with the nurses, and demanded that her new nickname be "Sassy."

On Friday, the 17th, Vanessa and I went to our older son's graduation. Terry graduated second in his class, and received the Kiwanis award. On Saturday, while Vicky was in the hospital, the rest of the family went with Terry to the Governor's mansion. The Governor awarded Terry salutatorian. During all of Vicky's treatment, Terry held a job, finished second in high school, kept up the house and yard, and helped watch the other two children. We were very proud of his accomplishments.

Vicky became very disoriented and weak for several days following chemotherapy. Vicky's kidney's were hurt by the chemotherapy, and started "leaking" the chemicals necessary for blood pressure control. Sodium bicarbonate was given orally to control blood pressure, but Vicky was not able to keep anything in her stomach. A blue tub was a common icon for all of the kids on the cancer ward. Vicky looked into the bottom of the tub every time her stomach erupted. Sometimes she didn't make the tub. Sodium bicarbonate was added to the IV along with antibiotics. On Monday, May 20, sodium bicarbonate levels started falling again which indicated the beginning of an infection. Vicky was transferred to PICU on the 21st because of degrading blood chemistry. Vanessa and I moved into the Ronald McDonald house as soon as there was an opening. Our chores this time required us to keep the paper towels in the kitchens stocked.

On May 22, a donor-directed blood drive was conducted at my work. Twenty-two units of whole blood were collected for Vicky. The blood was separated into the three basic parts of red blood, platelets, and plasma. The blood products were stored at Children's hospital for Vicky's use.

For the next two days increasing levels of blood pressure control were required, and Vicky remained stable. On Thursday, a CT scan of the abdomen was negative for infections allowing one of the antibiotics to be removed, which had bad side effects for the kidneys. It was obvious that an infection was still in her body, and the only place left to look was in the lungs. Vicky begged not to look in her lungs. Vanessa and I were sent out of the room. Vicky was sedated and placed on the ventilator. While turning Vicky over in this sedated condition, her rectum tore open. One of the side effects of one of the chemotherapy drugs was cracked skin. Four units of platelets and two units of red blood cells were required immediately. The doctor was very concerned about the possibility of bacteria in the colon going directly into the open wound. We were glad the donor directed blood products were on hand.

The sample from the lungs showed the presence of a fungus infection, and the presence of VRE (vancamycin resistant enteroccocus). VRE is staff bacteria that have built up immunity to all presently available antibiotics. With the presence of VRE and a tear in the rectum, the potential for VRE to infect the blood system existed. There are two antibiotics in development to treat VRE, but Children's Hospital was not able to obtain them. I contacted Senator Dale Bumpers and the White House for assistance. Only Senator Bumpers' office responded. One of the drug companies agreed to provide the antibiotic on a compassionate use basis, but only if an active VRE infection of the blood system was documented.

Antibiotics specific for Vicky's lung infection were started. Her lungs continued to get sicker, and more blood pressure control was required as the blood chemistry degraded. Vicky's blood counts dropped as a result of the chemotherapy. Red blood transfusions were required to maintain blood pressure, and platelets were required to stop bleeding. Over 20 units of blood products were transfused in two weeks. Vicky was at a state where she could wake up for short periods of time. She recognized everyone, and wanted lots of hugs and kisses. She responded to questions by shaking her head yes or no. We knew that her throat and rectum hurt a lot, and her right foot with an IV in it hurt also. An echogram of the heart showed damage caused by the chemotherapy. Vicky was now on a heart medication to force the heart to beat stronger.

One morning Vanessa and I noticed that the Children's Miracle Network Telethon was televised, and the local broadcast for Little Rock was coming from the Park Plaza Mall. Vanessa and I went to the mall for lunch to watch the telethon. The employees from our local Wal-Mart #66 were preparing to go on stage while we were watching, and we talked to them about Vicky's condition in the intensive care unit. When the Wal-Mart employees presented their check for the telethon, they mentioned that our son works for their store, and that his sister was in intensive care at Children's Hospital. Later in the afternoon, the hospital chaplain told us that he heard Vicky's name on the broadcast.

On June 5th Vicky did not know that I was in the room with her. She was reaching up into the air for something. When I asked if someone else was in the room, she nodded yes. I went through a list of names to find out who she thought was in the room with her: dad, mom, doctor, nurse, brother, sister, pastor, Jesus. At the name of Jesus, she nodded yes very strongly. My heart almost exploded as I asked if Jesus had come to take her home—she did not respond. I then asked if Jesus had come to heal her and again a strong yes. For the first time I believed that Vicky was going to survive. Vicky and I prayed together for Jesus to heal her. Following the prayer, Vicky mouthed "he healed me." I asked her if Jesus had indeed healed her, and she smiled and nodded yes. I wrote three names on a piece of paper—Victoria, Vicky, and Sassy. I asked Vicky what name she wants to be called by. From now on her nickname is "Sassy"—a name well deserved.

Going back to intensive care on life support was a great stress on Vanessa and I. Knowing how long it took to recover, knowing that chemotherapy needed to continue, knowing that radiation treatments were coming up soon, knowing how long it took to learn to walk again, and not knowing if Vicky would survive got to me. My chest and arm started hurting, and I did not sleep or rest. John, the chaplain at the hospital, noticed the problem, and helped to focus on my emotional needs. Following visits to the doctor, it was determined that the cause of my pain was stress.

I found help for this situation in Psalm 73. David's feelings and emotions in this Psalm were the same ones I experienced with Vicky's second time on the ventilator. Verse 1 truthfully states that God is good to those who are pure in heart. I rested in this knowledge, but the shock of the ventilator shook my foundation of faith, as it did David in verse 2. Verse 14 states that the difficulty lasted all day long, and it was there every morning. Verse 16 talks about pondering this difficulty day and night to try and understand what was going on. It troubled me all the time. Then, as verse 17 states, I came to the Lord, and I came to understanding. I found God teaching me the basics of sin, sickness, healing, and comfort.

On June 8, Children's Hospital sponsored a cancer convention and a survivor's picnic. At the convention, Vanessa and I learned about the history of childhood cancer, and the future of childhood cancer. Several survivors spoke at the end, and gave us hope for the future. I took video of Doctors Stine and Becton, and others, getting pies thrown in their faces by the cancer survivors. The picnic was a wonderful break away from PICU.

Saturday, June 15, Vicky left the intensive care unit after 26 days. While in the intensive care unit she was placed on a special airbed to prevent bedsores. Because of the strength Vicky developed in the final days of her stay in intensive care, she was allowed to go to the floor in her wheel chair. Her bed was sent to the 3rd floor without her in it. For Vanessa and I this was a major victory. Several people from the church came to visit Vicky, and were able to cheer her on as she transferred from the intensive care unit to her room. Vicky was presented with balloons and pajamas. Vicky wanted to change into the Tasmanian short set right away because "Taz" has her "Sassy" attitude.

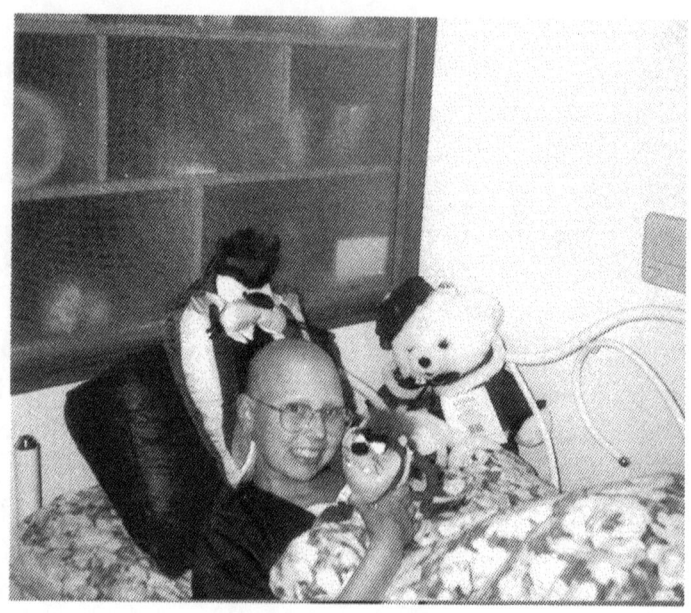

Vicky at home with Taz and her Taz pillow.

ANGELS ALL AROUND

Later in the evening, Vicky saw two angels in her room. She stated that, "The angels came to tell her that she was going to walk out of the hospital, and teach Sunday school again." I could not see them, but I could feel a calming presence. On Sunday, Vicky stated that "20 angels came to her room." She saw clouds in the ceiling, and the words "Healing and no more sickness." written on the clouds. The 20 angels told Vicky that, "100 legions of angels were on their way to watch over her." On Monday, June 17, Vicky said, "The 100 legions of angels arrived and took her up into heaven. There, she saw and heard the youth of our church praying for her healing." She said, "It was wonderful. The clouds of heaven and the hand of God stayed in her room all day." On Tuesday, Vicky had her bone scan. She was feeling so good, that the technicians were able to do the CT scans and X-rays also. When Vicky returned to her room she noticed that the number of angels had doubled to 200 legions. Vicky was feeling so good that she gave her nurses a "Sassy" time the rest of the day. Vicky said that being bossy makes people do things, but sassy invites people to do things. Vanessa and I told the stories of angels to our pastor and his wife. Sister Sheila asked us to record the stories. I tape recorded Vicky talking about the angels. While I was recording, Vicky said, "Jesus is on the wall." She recorded all of the words Jesus spoke to her. The tape was played at church for all of the people to hear.

On Wednesday and Thursday, Vicky had several scans. The results of the bone scan showed two possible new sites of cancer activity, but the MRI scans were negative. The scan of the left shoulder showed the soft tissue tumor to be at 50 percent of the original mass, and half of it was dead. On Friday, Vicky had a new IV port implanted and a bone marrow biopsy. This new port did not stick out of the skin like the other two. This one was under the skin. Vicky liked this type of port because it did not have to be cleaned and covered every day. On Monday, June 24, the doctor informed us that the bone marrow biopsy was normal, and there was no secondary cancer as a result of the chemotherapy.

Vicky wanted her back and feet massaged with lotion. I rubbed the breakdown spots of Vicky's back, and then massaged her feet. The breakdown spots felt like rocks under the skin. Vicky needed to use the bathroom, and as she stepped on the floor, her lotioned feet stated sliding. Vicky could have easily been hurt, but she looked so funny with both feet going in different directions. The nurse and I held Vicky up, but she was mad that I was laughing. As a result, I was not allowed to lotion her feet anymore. The nurse told Vicky that she needed to start wearing socks with grips on the bottoms.

Tuesday, June 25, Vicky, her nurse Rhonda, and I rode to Central Arkansas Radiation Technical Institute (CARTI) in the ambulance named, "Angel 2." At CARTI we learned that Vicky would receive 7 weeks of radiation to her left shoulder. The total integrated dose would be 5,500 Rads which is a lot of energy. A Rad is a standard measure of energy imparted in air by the radiation. Later in the evening Vicky said, "12 angels came into her room, and one of them was Gabriel. Each one was wearing a crown and blowing a horn. They were playing Amazing Grace." Vicky said, "some of the angels went with us on the ambulance to CARTI."

Vicky started making drawings of her experiences with the angels in her room. There is the angel Gabriel and a special 4-wing angel watching over 12 doves. Vicky laid out what heaven looked like, and she made a drawing of the crown Jesus was wearing. She put glitter on the crown, and stated that it represented all of the jewels that are in His crown. She drew pictures of friends and grandparents who were already in heaven.

Vicky said, "they came to comfort mom, dad, and others." There is a drawing of Jesus, and another of Satan being defeated by Gabriel. It was nice to know that Vicky had friends in high places looking after her.

Wednesday, June 26, Vicky walked to the door of her room using her walker. She was able to get up with her walker and use the bedside toilet. The doctor told Vicky that if she could walk 50 feet, and eat well, she could leave the hospital the following Tuesday. Vicky was so proud of herself. She ordered some french onion dip, and started in with a bag of potato chips. The next round of chemotherapy was started in the afternoon.

Greg Adams, with social services, placed Vicky and the family in an apartment in West Little Rock for the 7 weeks of radiation at CARTI. The apartment is called "Open Arms." Vicky was so excited. She planned on going shopping, and expected me to pay for lots of cloths. Vicky left the hospital on July 2. We left the hospital with a feeding tube and a pump. Each night Vicky received 12 hours of a high protein liquid through a feeding tube going down her nose. Again Vanessa and I had to be trained in the use and care of the pump and feed tube.

On Friday, July 5, Vicky went back into Children's Hospital because of low blood pressure, and received 2 units of red blood and 2 units of platelets. The effects of the chemotherapy caused the blood counts to drop. Vicky stayed two nights, and went back to the apartment in Little Rock. She left the hospital in her wheel chair.

"I know it has been a struggle, but I know how tough you are. Keep fighting, and someday I'll get to see you walk out of here."
Mike Binns, PICU Respiratory Therapist

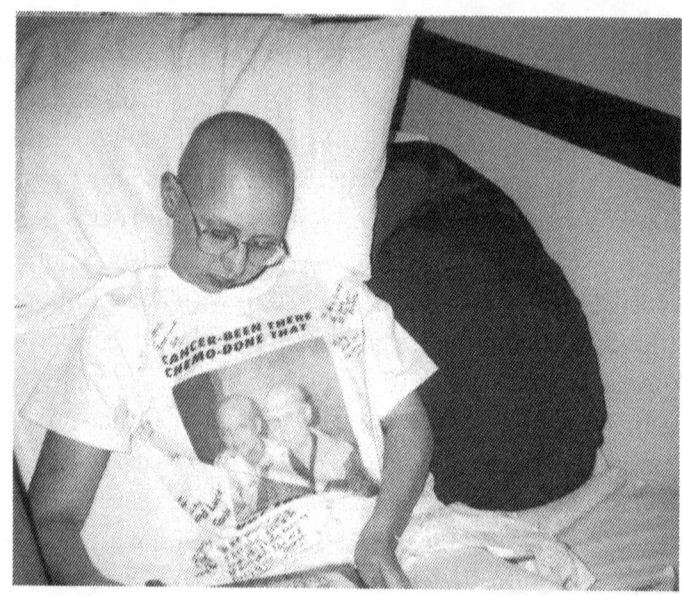

Vicky drawing. Her T-shirt has her and Kara on the front.

A Miracle in Motion

At the apartment, there were 13 steps from the parking lot to the side walk. Each day Vicky climbed the stairs, and was quickly gaining strength. On the 15th of July, Vicky was able to climb the stairs by herself. She started using her walker for all of the short trips to the radiation center and around the apartment. The wheel chair was used for trips to the mall, Wal-Mart, and the grocery store. She was eating so well that the feeding tube was removed.

Vicky was placed on a bed at CARTI to mark the locations for radiation. The computer used to focus the radiation on the cancer, and keep it away from the lung, fabricated a special lead mold. Lasers marked the spots and then black permanent markers were used to put an X at several locations. Vicky felt no sensation of any kind during the radiation treatments.

From the time Vicky received her blood and platelet transfusions on the 5th of July, her red blood and platelet counts remained constant, but the white blood count was steadily dropping. It was believed that the effects of radiation were keeping counts from going up. On the 23rd of July radiation was stopped in order to help the blood counts go up. Vicky started the white cell growth factor injections on July 23. Vicky's counts started up, and the growth factor was stopped on August 1. On August 2 Vicky went back into Children's hospital for 3 more units of red blood. The following day Vicky walked out of the hospital by herself for the first time since going into the hospital in January. The angels that came to visit Vicky stated that she would walk out of the hospital, and teach Sunday school again. Part of the message had come true.

On August 6, Vicky went to Westside High School in Johnson County, and registered for her senior year. Vicky was also enrolled in Pulaski County for homebound schooling while receiving radiation. Vicky was expected to graduate with her senior class. The homework that piled up while Vicky was in intensive care was completed. She started building an AM/FM radio provided by the VoTech Vicky attended last year. Vicky was excited about school, and was looking forward to going to the prom. She found her a black prom dress, and a date. Vicky stated that I was the only date good enough to take her to the prom. I chose to agree with her.

Later in the evening, Vanessa started having chest pain, and difficulty breathing. She stated that she was scared of how she was feeling. I rushed her to the emergency room. It was determined that stress was the cause of the problems. Vanessa was sent back home.

On August 8, Arkansas Children's Dreams and the Arkansas Travelers ball team held a benefit at Ray Winder Field in Little Rock. Vicky received an autographed baseball, and was invited up to the press box. Sassy climbed all the way to the top of the stadium. While up there, her name was flashed all over the scoreboard. Sassy climbed all the way down where she ordered three icees, a coke, and popcorn.

Each blood test showed the white count dropping again, and the red blood and platelet counts remaining constant. Since August 9, Vicky's white blood count dropped so low that she could easily get an infection. Vanessa and I kept Vicky away from crowds, and we stayed in the apartment in Little Rock until all blood counts were high enough for the next round of chemotherapy. The oncology doctors believed that the lingering effect of chemotherapy given June 26–28 along with radiation was responsible for the low blood counts. They also believed that the medications used to control seizures over stimulated the kidneys, and were responsible for the periods of chemical induced commas.

On Saturday, August 10, Vicky laid down her walker. She went to the medical supply store and purchased a cane. She found the cane much easier to use than the walker. On Monday, August 12, her wheel chair was turned in. The growth factor injections for the white blood cell growth was restarted on August 13, and radiation to the shoulder was also restarted.

Vicky enjoyed walking to the pool at the apartment. The buoyancy of the water made it easy for her to walk around the pool. The management of the apartments had a "dawg daze at the water'n hole." Vicky had so much fun meeting all of the people from the apartments. She won a $10.00 gift certificate to the Macaroni Grill as a door prize.

The door prize was used to celebrate Vicky's birthday. The last time we were in the macaroni grill, Vicky could not eat. This time she ate her meal. The management presented Vicky a birthday cake, and sang "happy birthday" in Italian.

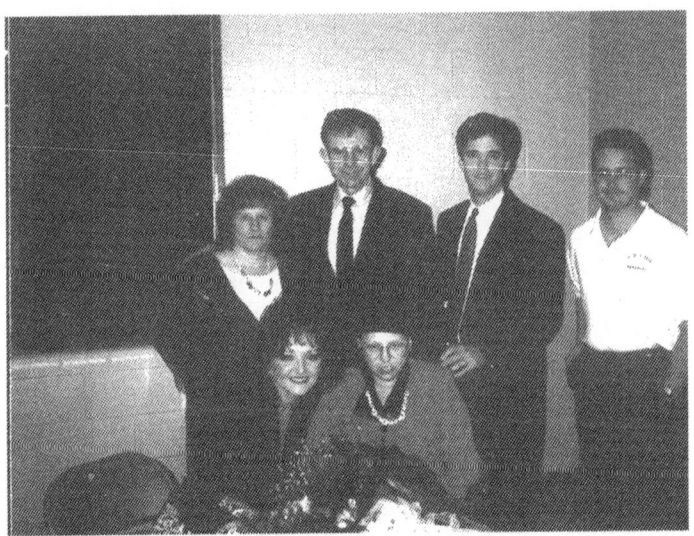

Vanessa, Tom, and Vicky meeting with Karen Wheaton. The TLC representatives are on the right.

The ABCs of VRE

Bacteria resistant to the antibiotic "vancomycin" was first reported in 1988. Studies were conducted at 97 centers in 1992, and 23 percent of the centers reported the presence of vancomycin resistant enteroccocus (VRE). By March 1994, 61 percent of the sites reported VRE. The 1995 Center for Disease Control (CDC) guidelines for limiting the spread of VRE in hospitals require prompt implementation of measures to control spread of the organism. (Report on Pediatric Infectious Diseases, Volume 6, Number 2, February 1996, pages 5-6).

Vanessa and I reviewed articles from the Children's Hospital library, including CDC recommendations for a VRE isolation policy. The tenacity of VRE presented in these articles generated immediate fear for Vicky's future. The infection control department at Children's Hospital was contacted to discuss every possible aspect of VRE. It was apparent that the hospital was concerned about other patients, but there were unanswered questions about VRE and the general public. Vanessa and I contacted the "Hospital Infection Control Physician" on call at CDC. We were informed that the community at large was not at risk, however health care workers entering the home would have to practice isolation to protect other patients in the community.

A training session was held at Children's Hospital on August 20 to discuss VRE. The church pastor, home health nurses, Vicky, and her family were present. Also present at the training was the social worker, oncology department, pathology department, and the nursing department. Dr. Terry Yamauchi was the mediator. Dr. Yamauchi is the

Professor and Vice-Chairman of Pediatrics Infectious Diseases Division at Children's Hospital. He also works for the University at Arkansas for Medical Sciences (UAMS), and teaches at CDC. He was instrumental in the development of the CDC guidelines for VRE.

There are several issues that need to be addressed early on for any family dealing with VRE. The first item we discussed was how VRE is created. From January 12 until January 17, Vicky was administered antibiotics for a fever, and between January 17 and February 18, she was in PICU with an infection. It is important to understand that antibiotics are effective for bacteria only. Pathogens can include bacteria, virus, yeast, and mold and each is controlled in a specific manner. Until the mold in Vicky's lungs was identified around the 22nd of January, bacteria were considered a possible pathogen. And as long as Vicky's white count remained low, a bacterial infection was likely.

The second item we covered was how bacteria respond to antibiotics. Enteroccocus bacteria live in the colon, and are part of the digestive process. When antibiotics are administered, the population of bacteria in the colon decreases. Vicky was administered first, second, and third generation antibiotics in an attempt to bring an end to the infection. The bacteria in the colon responded to the antibiotics and developed immunity to all of the antibiotics. This is where the VRE in Vicky came from. Since enteroccocus bacteria are normally in the colon, it is not considered a pathogen until it invades the body. It was on April 1st, while Vicky's white count was low, when the VRE of the colon entered into the body as a pathogen. The VRE never caused an infection.

The third item we covered was why isolation was required in the hospital. Isolation of the patient is required in order to prevent other "at risk" patients from becoming colonized with VRE. The "at risk" patient is a person without an immune system. These patients are very much aware of their condition, and are concerned about catching any type of illness. The CDC guidelines for isolation assume that the patient with VRE cannot control their bowels, has open sores, and does not practice good hygiene. Under these conditions, VRE is easily transferred to health care workers who could then carry the bacteria to other patients. The room is sterilized each shift since VRE, like all bacteria, cannot live on dry surfaces. Coughing and sneezing are not a concern because VRE lives in the colon, not the airway unless VRE is a pathogen in the airway.

Once the patient is able to control his/her bowels, open sores are healed, and good hygiene is followed, the spread of VRE is highly unlikely. The patient can shake hands and even hug individuals without any concern of VRE. Individuals with a normal immune system do not have to be concerned with VRE. The normal forms of bacteria in their colon will prevent the VRE from colonizing.

It was noted that Vicky had never had a VRE blood infection while her white count was low. Vicky was admitted to PICU on three occasions, and VRE was never a contributor to any complications. It was also noted that there was a 99.9 percent chance that VRE would never cause an infection. Should a VRE blood infection ever occur, there are two antibiotics available for the treatment of VRE. The drugs are still in the development process, and would be administered under the "compassionate care" program. The hospital contacted the drug manufacturer, and I contacted my senator. I had obtained congressional intervention for Vicky to have access to these new drugs.

The CDC guidelines require two negative samples, taken two weeks apart, to declare the patient free of VRE. Vicky would not be tested for the absence of VRE until she had completed all chemotherapy. The hospital would take the conservative approach and continue to observe isolation requirements when Vicky was admitted to the hospital. Once chemotherapy was completed, and Vicky's normal immune system was restored, VRE was expected to go away on its own.

The expectation for Vicky, and the family, when attending church, or other community functions, was to use proper hygiene. The expectation for all immune suppressed individuals with low white blood counts, including Vicky, was to avoid contact with others. Live immunizations to infants, chicken pox, and the common cold virus are a much greater threat than VRE.

From 1988 to the present, the number of VRE cases has continued to increase. Some of the cases are from the use of antibiotics, and others by transfer from one patient to another by health care workers. A hospital directed isolation policy alone has not stopped the spread of VRE. A team approach using the CDC, hospital, patient, family, and community is required. The most powerful tool in this team has been education.

Everyone was pleased with the training. Our pastor relayed the information to the church. But, not everyone accepted the pastor's report. Teachers wanted to know if other students were at risk of dying. One family went so far as to demand that Vicky be thrown out of the church. Rumors traveled at speeds that seemed to exceed the speed of light. Vicky was heart broken when she learned that some in the church did not welcome her.

I had to go before the church board to defend Vicky. I wanted to lay aside my Christianity, but the greater need was Vicky. When all of the words were spoken it was obvious that fear of an unknown, such as VRE, ruled in peoples hearts. I agreed to keep Vicky away from people until Dr. Terry Yamauchi could come speak to the church.

Dr. Terry Yamauchi agreed to meet with our church on October 6 following concerns expressed by the members. Several church members had obtained the CDC guidelines, and assumed that they applied to the general public at all times.

Dr. Yamauchi pointed out that the CDC guidelines are benchmarks for the CDC to use to determine the effectiveness of controlling VRE. Dr. Yamauchi then stated specifically how VRE was transferred from one person to another.

VRE is called "bowel-hand-mouth" bacteria. The bacteria exist in the colon of the colonized patient. The hands can get contaminated after a bowel movement. If good hygiene is not followed, then the bacteria can be passed to another person. This other person has to get the bacteria into the mouth to become colonized with VRE. If either the patient or other person use proper hygiene, they stop the spread of VRE. VRE is not absorbed through the skin, and is not an airborne bacterium, and you cannot get it by kissing a colonized person.

Proper hygiene by everyone was the best way to stop the spread of VRE. Dr. Yamauchi explained everything to the church, and then took questions from the congregation. There were questions like "Can I eat in a restaurant after Vicky has been in it." And, "Can I sit in the same pew Vicky sat in."

In the end Vicky was allowed to freely come and go to church. But, one family refused to touch Vicky or anyone in my family. I was amazed at Vicky's attitude. She felt sorry for the family, and always prayed for them.

THE HALFWAY POINT

On August 23, radiation to the shoulder was completed, and the next round of chemotherapy was started on the 28th. Because of the low platelet count, the normal three days of chemotherapy was shortened to two days. On the 30th, Vicky needed 3 units of red blood cells, and on September 4 she needed two units of platelets, and three more units of red blood cells. The red blood helped to give Vicky back the energy the chemotherapy took away.

One evening Sassy left her cane in the car and started walking to the apartment without any assistance. Vicky was feeling good about herself. She liked showing off the amount of strength she was gaining in her legs and arms each day. Everyone was so proud of her efforts, and Vicky loved the attention she was getting. Each night, Vicky did exercises, including 100 curls with her right arm using a five-pound weight. She wanted to arm wrestle with the nurses the next time she went in the hospital.

Vicky's infection fighting white blood count dropped to zero, and the growth factor injections were restarted. We moved home on Saturday, September 7. We were thankful to the staff and management who provided the Open Arms apartment.

Vicky was able to ride the Children's Medical Service (CMS) van for the first time to Children's Hospital on September 11 for her check ups. Dr. Nicholas, the orthopedic surgeon, evaluated Vicky's shoulder. The muscles that rotate the arm outward and back were paralyzed. The muscle that lifted the arm up was also paralyzed. The tumor's rapid growth in the shoulder area was responsible for the damage. Dr. Nicholas noted that the bone was showing signs of healing. He could not detect any tumor masses in the shoulder area. It takes one billion cancer cells to make a mass large enough to be detected. Because the tumor did exist, chemotherapy would be continued long enough to kill all undetectable cancer cells.

Vicky also visited the oncology department. Her nose was bleeding, and a blood count showed her platelets low at four thousand. The kids learned to say the number was four and they knew that was a low number. Vicky received one unit of platelets before going home.

Vicky was feeling so good about the good report. On the way home she picked up the groceries to fix burritos. At home, Vicky cooked the meal all by herself and set the table. Vicky wanted her life and the family routine to return to normal. Vicky then ate half a burrito. Vanessa and I were left with doing dishes.

On the 15th of September Vicky turned 17 with a birthday party at the Lazy Earl's restaurant in Clarksville. Vicky invited her aunts and uncles, but none of them showed up. Vicky was not upset at all. She said, "they were the ones who missed out on a wonderful birthday party."

The next round of chemotherapy was started on September 25th, and lasted only three days. Cytoxan was given in place of iphosfamide. The liver breaks down Cytoxan while the kidneys break down iphosfamide. Vicky's kidneys could not handle anymore iphosfamide. On the 26th, Vicky needed three units of red blood. The side effects of cytoxan are hair loss, bladder irritation or hemorrhage, anemia, low blood counts, immunosuppression, water overload, sterility, lung scarring, increased skin pigmentation, loss of appetite, nausea, vomiting, sore mouth, diarrhea, gastrointestinal ulcers, and increased uric acid.

Vanessa's sister, Sheila, died at home of cancer on September 28. Vicky was very close to Aunt Sheila, and enjoyed talking to her. Vicky started to question if she would die of cancer like her aunt did. Vicky also wanted to know if she gave cancer to Aunt Sheila. Vicky's enthusiasm gave way to sadness.

On October 2nd, Vicky was very tired, and could not eat or drink. I convinced Vicky that she needed the feed tube to keep from getting too sick. I inserted the feeding tube to start the liquid feeds. Vicky took a deep breath before I inserted the tube. She started gagging instantly. I cleaned up the mess and tried again. Vicky signaled me with her hand to stop when the tube was half way in. She took deep breaths, but she could not stop the nausea. Vicky asked to rest a few minutes before trying again. This time I did not stop when Vicky signaled to stop. I pushed the tube all the way in and held it in place as Vicky emptied her stomach. The tube came up her stomach and out her mouth. And I pulled the tube back out. I let Vicky rest an hour before trying again. This time the tube stayed in place. During the night Vicky said that she heard angels singing "Amazing Grace," and that she kept hearing Aunt Sheila talking. Vicky did not rest well all night.

In the morning, Vicky was nauseated, and spit up the feeding tube. With the tube in her nose and out her mouth, there was a constant gag reflex. I removed the feed tube, and noticed that Vicky's mouth was coated with blood. We packed our bags and headed for the emergency room at Children's Hospital.

Vicky's blood count showed the platelet level lower than we had ever seen it at 2.0. Her blood pressure was low, and she started to run a fever. Vicky was given a liter of fluids by IV, and admitted to room 3129 for antibiotics and two units of platelets. Vicky asked the doctor if the nurse could put in a feed tube. The doctor agreed and the feed tube was inserted. Vicky asked Mom and I to leave the room while the tube was inserted.

Vicky asked to talk with the chaplain, John. She was very upset at the loss of Aunt Sheila, and the idea that she had cancer also. Vanessa and I left the room while John and Vicky talked. John spoke with Vanessa and me afterwards and said that Vicky was feeling much better about the loss of her Aunt. Vicky called our pastor's wife, Sister Sheila, but Vicky was too exhausted to hold a conversation. Sister Sheila prayed while I held the phone to Vicky's ear. Vicky was given three units of red blood, and her energy started to return.

Blood cultures showed two types of bacteria in the blood stream. The protocol for these two bacteria required ten days of antibiotics. Vicky's stomach was plagued with nausea because of the chemotherapy. She did not take any food or liquids by mouth all week. Nourishment was by liquids through a feed tube through the nose, and into the intestinal tract. The renal panel (blood test) results were the best they had been since starting chemotherapy, and Vicky gained strength each day.

Red blood counts continued to drop, and on October 4, Vicky received three more units of red blood. On October 7, she received a unit of platelets. Vicky's platelet level continued to drop, and on October 11, the injection site for the white blood cell growth factor bled into the surrounding area. Vicky was scheduled to go home on the morning of October 12, but Vicky requested one more unit of platelets before being released. Vicky liked to wear shorts and she did not want any bruises on her legs.

Vicky was feeling so good that she baked a birthday cake for Mom's birthday on October 14. Vicky went to Wal-Mart, and picked up birthday and Christmas presents for friends and family. She spent the afternoon working on homework, and doing physical therapy.

Vicky went back to Clinic 3 on Wednesday, October 16, for a CT scan and MRI of the left shoulder. The tumor mass was mainly scar tissue now. When all of the chemotherapy and radiation treatments are over, she could decide if she wanted the scar tissue removed.

Vicky started giving her own growth factor injections. She also took charge of her daily medications. She asked me for an exercise bike and I found one at a garage sell. Vicky's left arm was gaining more motion due to the physical therapy. Vicky found it enjoyable riding the bike and doing her exercises. I started to wonder if Vicky had a crush on her doctors or therapist. Vicky denied any such notion, but her smile and eyes told a different story.

When Vicky went back to Children's Hospital for the next round of treatment a tornado came through Little Rock in the evening. All of the kids were moved out into the hallways. Vicky's bed was next to Kara's bed. Kara was 17 years old, and had Ewing's sarcoma also. The two girls immediately started sharing stories about their cancer and boyfriends. Vicky and Kara became best friends through the storms of life.

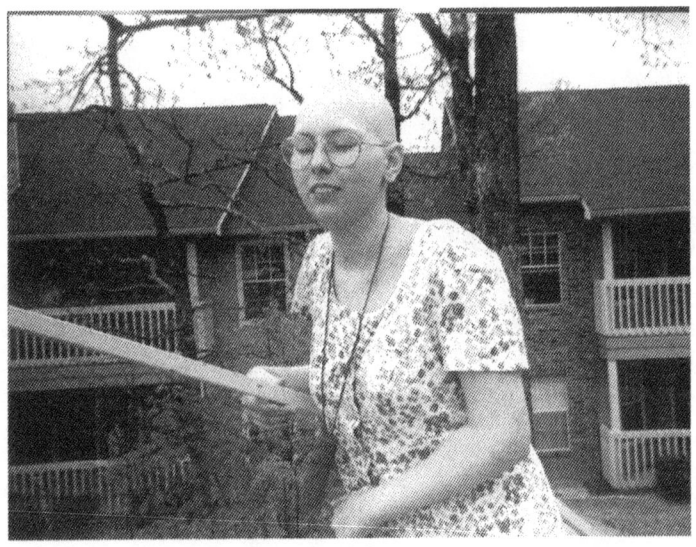

Vicky is climbing the steps at the Open Arms apartment.

Nurse Abuse

Vicky's self-esteem constantly improved because of the social interaction with her nurses. Vicky started sharing her book during her October 3 to 12 stay at Children's Hospital. Several nurses looked to make sure they were not named within the pages. Vicky immediately decided to add a section describing the many times she pushed back at the nurses, as they would encourage her to fight. Therefore this section is dedicated to the Hip Police, Boots, the Boss, Trashy, and all of the other nurses Vicky come in contact with.

In order to be balanced in life, an individual must have a balance in his/her physical growth, spiritual growth, mental growth, and social growth. For Vicky, these areas were greatly modified because of cancer and chemotherapy. Physical and occupational therapists helped with the physical growth. The homebound teacher and hospital teacher helped with the mental growth. The social worker, chaplain, and our pastor helped with spiritual growth. Vicky's social world was greatly modified because of her suppressed immune system and VRE. As a result, the majority of Vicky's social circle was made up of nurses. This chapter describes this social circle where Vicky was encouraged to build a fighting spirit. Vicky wanted to nickname this fighting spirit "nurse abuse."

On one occasion Vicky called her nurse Rhonda over the intercom. Vicky told Rhonda that she needed help. Vicky had her cow bean bag hidden under the covers. Vicky waited a moment, and then threw the cow at Rhonda and scared her. Vicky laughed with Rhonda each time she came into the room because Rhonda would ask where the cow was.

On another occasion Janet came into Vicky's room to transfuse platelets. Vicky was busy painting. When Janet turned away, Vicky painted Janet's isolation gown. When Janet noticed what happened, she told Vicky to just wait. Janet grabbed the paintbrush, and painted the top of Vicky's head. Vicky tried to wipe the paint off with her pillowcase, but it just painted more of her head. Vanessa had to get Vicky a wet paper towel. Vicky promised to get even.

On one occasion while at CARTI, Vicky picked up a rubber glove that was easy to blow up into a balloon. Vicky then painted the glove in the likeness of a punk rocker, and named it Rhonda. Vicky showed it to all of the nurses and doctors before showing Rhonda.

On the way back from Disneyland, Vicky found a card for her nurse, Rhonda. There was a cute girl standing in a trashcan holding a rose. Vicky gave Rhonda the nickname "trashy" because of that card. Vicky told Rhonda that her theme song was the one about "liking women a little on the trashy side"

On another day Rhonda brought some ice into Vicky's room. When Rhonda turned around, Vicky took a piece of the ice and put it down Rhonda's shirt. Vicky laughed hard when Rhonda jumped.

When Vicky was just out of PICU for the first time, she could barely move around in the bed. Vicky had three bedsores on her back, and the chemotherapy had irritated her bottom. Everyone was encouraging Vicky to lay on her sides. One of the night nurses threatened to bring in a whistle and blow it each time Vicky was suppose to change sides. Every time the nurse would come in the room, she would roll Vicky to the other side. Vicky nicknamed her the "hip police."

One evening one of the male nurses gave Vicky her injection in the leg, and Vicky thought it hurt too much. Vicky told her nurses the next day, and the nurses encouraged Vicky to get him back. Vicky pinched Andrew on the bottom the next night. Andrew wanted to know what he did to deserve such treatment. Vicky said she liked him.

The nurses continued to encourage Vicky to move her feet, especially when there was breakdown of the skin. Vicky would kick at the nurses and tell them to just go away. One day one of the nurses started kicking back. Vicky and Boots made a game of seeing who would get kicked first. Vicky said it was much more fun kicking nurses than getting kicked out of church.

TOO MANY PILLS

O n Sunday morning, October 20, the family had a scare when Vicky fell onto her left side. Vicky tripped over toys at the end of Stacy's bed while getting dressed for church. There was the sound of someone falling, and then Vanessa cried out for me to come quickly. Vicky's left knee quickly swelled just below the kneecap, and she had a lot of pain. Vanessa and I were scared that Vicky might have broken her left arm that was treated with radiation. But, Vicky said that her arm was fine. There was a lot of bruising to the knee because of low platelets. I wrapped Vicky's knee in an ace bandage while big tears were dripping from her cheeks. Vicky's pain let up, and she asked to go on to church. Vicky sat quietly through Sunday school, but her knee started to hurt her again. During the morning service Vicky went into the nursery, and put her feet up while sitting in a rocking chair. After the service Vicky wanted to have her knee x-rayed for her own peace of mind, but Vicky had invited the pastor and his wife out to lunch before Sunday school. Vicky wanted spaghetti without any meat at Pizza Hut. The pastor was not fond of pizza, so Vicky talked him into eating the spaghetti with her. Vicky was overjoyed to have a chance to do something for our pastor and his wife. Vicky kept her leg propped up during the meal, and never complained of any pain. More than anything else, Vicky wanted to spend time talking with Sister Sheila.

There is a local hospital where Vicky's knee could be x-rayed, but the hospital is not a preferred provider on the family insurance. I drove the 30 miles to the emergency room while Vicky lay back in the seat. The x-ray showed that none of Vicky's bones were broken, and a blood test showed that she did not need a platelet transfusion. Vicky felt comfortable going back home with an ice pack on her knee. Around 10:00 p.m. Vicky's left shoulder started to hurt, and she asked Vanessa and I to come look. There was swelling at the socket joint on the outside of the arm. Vicky was in tears, and asked for morphine to control the pain. At 5:00 a.m. Vicky woke me, and asked for an ice pack on her left shoulder. Vicky was afraid that the radiation to her shoulder made it easy to break a bone in her shoulder. Vicky was scared, and wanted her shoulder x-rayed for her own peace of mind again. Vanessa and I took Vicky to her pediatrician and had the shoulder x-rayed. None of the bones were broken. We now had experience knowing that Vicky could take a fall without causing any major injuries. But we did all we could to keep the floors at the house clear for Vicky. Vicky was always the first one to scold one of her brothers or sister if anything was left on a floor.

Vicky was able to go with the family to Fort Smith for the first time since being diagnosed with cancer. Her younger brother, Windle, had a scheduled appointment with his neurologist. Vicky's neurologist, Doctor James Barry, was able to check Vicky while she was at the clinic. When Vicky weighed in, the nurse noted that Vicky had lost 41 pounds from her last visit a year ago. Doctor Barry contacted home health, and asked for a Phenobarbital level to see if it was at a minimum therapeutic level.

Home health nurses came out to the house for Vicky's blood work on the 24th. I called children's hospital in the afternoon for the results to see if it was time for the next round of chemotherapy. Vicky's platelet level was 84, and the level needed to be above 100. Vicky's potassium level was very low. Vicky was already taking one potassium pill four times a day. The oncologist told me to increase the dosage for potassium up to two pills four times a day. The neurologist, Doctor Barry, called later in the afternoon, and changed Vicky's Phenobarbital dosage from three pills a day to four pills a day. Doctor Barry wanted a minimum therapeutic level, which should prevent seizures. Vicky was not happy at all about taking five more pills each day.

On the evening of the 26th I was joking around with Vicky at the dinner table. Vicky did not like anyone to mess with her bald head. I figured that if Janet could get away with it so could I. I used my finger to paint the top of Vicky's head with some mustard and strawberry ice cream syrup. Vicky exploded with fury, and dumped her plate of spaghetti all over my head. The other kids were doubled over with laughter as Vicky wiped her head. I went into the bathroom to clean up, and noticed one of Vicky's pills next to the trash can. A quick search found several rounds of pills wadded up in toilet paper in the trash can. I returned to the dinner table, and asked Vicky if she was taking all of her pills. She said that she was. I showed the retrieved pills to Vicky, and asked her why the pills were not taken. With the same furry about painting her head, Vicky said "I am getting tired of taking so many pills all the time." Vicky then ran to her bed and started crying. Buried in the sobs were accusations that no one understands what it is like to have cancer. I prayed with Vicky until she calmed down. The sobs soon subsided. Vicky and I used the list of medications to talk about each pill, and what it did for her body. Vicky agreed to start taking all of her pills again. Her tear soaked eyes fixed on mine, and then she warned me not to touch her head again. She laughed as she threw her pillow in my face.

Sunday, October 27, was the best day Vicky had since being diagnosed with cancer. She was excited about going to church and took extra steps to prepare her long wig. Vicky got the response she expected. Most of the people told Vicky that she looked beautify while one family did all they could to avoid her. Without any prompting, Vicky ate each meal, her fluid intake was super, and she swallowed all of her medications on time. Vicky started right in with her homework right after church. When it came time for me to help with Vicky's physical therapy, she asked to do more repetitions on each exercise than what was required. Vicky was in charge of life and it showed in her deep blue eyes. All of her eye lashes and eyebrows were gone, but her eyes were full of life.

On Monday morning Vicky woke up with the munchies. But when she ate sweet pickles and cream cheese, her stomach was upset. Vicky needed a pill for the nausea. Vicky called her Uncle Marvin for some of his famous macaroni and cheese. He promised to bring it over for lunch. The home health nurse arrived, and drew Vicky's blood. When I called for the results, the red blood count was less than 6.0. The kids with cancer learned that this was a low number. Children's Hospital scheduled Vicky to transfuse two units of red blood the next day in the day medicine clinic. Between lunch and dinner, Vicky snacked on four large bowls of Uncle Marvin's macaroni and cheese.

On Tuesday morning, Vanessa and Vicky rode the CMS van to children's hospital for the red blood transfusion. I took Stacy to day care on the way to work, and Terry placed Windle on the bus for school. Vicky's blood counts were checked at the hospital, and her platelet level was 177. Vicky was scheduled to start chemotherapy the next day. Vanessa called me, and asked to stay the night in Little Rock. Debbie Cole, from my work, picked up Stacy from day care, and planned to keep her for a few days. Stacy and Debbie's daughter, Georgia, were best of friends. I left work early and drove to Little Rock. I picked up Vicky and Vanessa at the hospital, and went to a motel. Terry watched Windle at home after school. Vanessa called Terry, and asked him to pack her a suitcase.

The next round of chemotherapy was started on October 30th. After Terry put Windle on the school bus, he placed Mom and Vicky's luggage on the CMS van. Vicky was admitted to room 3139, in the bone marrow transplant area, because all other rooms on the cancer ward were full. Kara Travis was in the hospital for her chemotherapy and heard that Vicky was being admitted. Before Vicky was connected to the I.V. pump, she and Kara visited in Kara's room. The two caught up on their activities since their last visit. Kara then gave a present to Vicky.

Vicky was still in the hospital for Halloween. Doctor Nicholas visited each of his patients and presented them a special piece of candy. Vicky asked Mom to put her candy next to the stuffed animals. The stuffed animals were one of Vicky's treasures. Each one had a story to tell. The candy deserved the same recognition. The kids in the hospital were encouraged to dress up for Halloween. Vicky dressed up like a doctor with one of the doctor's lab coats and a stethoscope. The nurses and staff made Halloween so much fun with lots of activities. Vicky painted some pumpkins, but Sassy's favorite activity was arguing with her nurses. Vanessa and I had a chance to meet Kara's mom for the first time. She was just as overwhelmed with cancer and chemotherapy as we were in the beginning. The only way to know the stress Kara's mom was facing was to be in the same situation.

Vicky was discharged at 10:30 at night on the first of November. Vicky wanted so much to stay the night in the hospital simply because she was tired. But, insurance would not pay for the night unless it was medically necessary. Vanessa, Vicky, and I went to a motel for the night.

Vicky said she wanted some hash browns from Denny's for breakfast the next morning but Vicky did not eat or drink anything. Vicky finally promised to drink her small glass of Dr. Pepper if I would buy her a Reba McEntire CD. The drink went down, and Vicky went to Wal-Mart in Little Rock. Vicky also wanted to shop at the Wal-Mart at home in Clarksville. Looking at clothes, and visiting with friends made Vicky feel much better. After getting to the house, Vicky wanted to go out to dinner with Terry. Vicky did not eat very much at all, but she and Terry talked at length about guns and cars. Vicky wanted so much to talk with everyone. The injections to increase the white blood count were started, and at bedtime Vicky gave her own injection.

On Sunday morning Vicky did her best to dress up and put on her makeup. Vicky enjoyed it so much when the people at church noticed how good she looked. She also knew that one family would never accept her as being normal. The whole family went to Sunday school and church. The family went to Russellville after church to pick up Stacy at Debbie's home. Vicky was acting "Sassy," and wanted some Mexican food. Sassy's appetite for Mexican food was amazing. We went to a Mexican restaurant in Russellville where Sassy ate refried beans, chips and dip, a cheese enchilada, and a bean burrito. After lunch Vicky and I went to J.C. Penny to look for some clothes. She found a hat and vest for her Christmas outfit. I found a pretty long blue dress for one of Vicky's Christmas gifts. Vicky's grandpa in California called in the evening, and spoke for a long time with Vicky. Grandpa and Grandma were planning on coming out to visit. If possible they would come around Thanksgiving.

Vicky paged me at work Monday morning after the home health nurse took her blood. She wanted me to meet her and Vanessa for lunch at a Mexican restaurant. Vicky did not eat very much. I called the hospital for Vicky's blood counts. Her blood counts were low, and she was scheduled for a red blood transfusion Thursday morning.

Because of the early time of Vicky's transfusion, and the fact that I was getting very tired, the family went to Little Rock Wednesday evening. On the way out of town Windle was left with the pastor at the church. After church, Windle went home with the Youth Pastor's family. When Terry got off of work, he picked up Windle and took him home. Vanessa, Vicky, Stacy, and I checked into a motel and then went to another Mexican restaurant for dinner. Vicky's food volume and liquid volume was very low for her. I considered the eating and drinking problems to be a combination of low blood counts and the side effects of chemotherapy.

Vicky checked in at the day clinic where she was scheduled for two units of red blood. I had started graphing Vicky's red blood counts, platelet counts, and white counts. The graph for Vicky's platelet level indicated that Vicky should also get some platelets. I requested a blood test to verify my assumption. The test results showed Vicky's platelet level at 8, and falling. I took the test results and graphs to Doctor

Becton. The doctor agreed with my projections, and ordered two units of platelets. This made me feel good about my efforts to predict Vicky's need for blood product transfusions and the length of time that Vicky's white count would be at or near zero. Vicky received a Vincristine chemotherapy boost along with her transfusions. When I returned to Vicky's room, her morning and noon pills were gone, but very little of her coke was gone. Vicky claimed that she took the pills, but a search of the trash can in the bathroom showed a different story. Vicky refused to answer why she did not take her pills.

On the way home Vicky wanted to eat some mashed potatoes at Kentucky Fried Chicken. She ate about three bites and would not drink. Vicky had less than four ounces to drink all day long. A large mouth sore had developed, and it hurt Vicky to move her mouth even to speak. Vicky asked for the feed tube to be inserted when she got home. Vicky got sick when the feed tube was inserted, and she threw up a large volume. I was getting comfortable inserting the feed tube, but it still hurt me to watch Vicky's eyes fill with tears. I started liquid feeds, and ground up her medications. Each time I gave Vicky her medications; she would get nauseated, and threw up the contents of her stomach. I was getting frustrated with having to clean up the mess.

Vicky had trouble sleeping during the night because of bad dreams about the death of Aunt Sheila. Vicky woke me up during the night and asked me to stay in her room for a while. Her pillow was soaked with tears. I prayed for Vicky, and she went back to sleep. Vicky's energy was completely gone in the morning, and she needed help getting out of bed. A home health nurse came out to the house Friday morning and obtained Vicky's blood for lab tests. The nurse noticed the large mouth sore in the left side of Vicky's mouth. I called Children's Hospital later in the day for the results of the blood tests. When I plotted the results, I noticed that Vicky would need red blood and platelet transfusions by Wednesday. Vicky already had an appointment at Children's Hospital for Wednesday. Vicky was scared about how weak she was. She understood that her counts were low and was comforted knowing she would get the needed transfusions on Wednesday. Sister Sheila came out to visit with Vicky, and left some work to keep her occupied. Vicky was given a set of large posters and markers for use in the next Sunday school quarter. Sister Sheila wanted Vicky to color these posters. The two talked for a long time and then prayed before Sister Sheila went home. Vicky did not want Sister Sheila to leave.

Vicky was a little more alert Saturday morning. Vicky got a bath, and got ready to go to her Aunt Paula's house for their son's birthday party. When Vicky arrived at Paula's house, several people were smoking. Vicky started choking and crying. The smokers went to the back of the house as soon as they noticed what the smoke was doing to Vicky. All Vicky had strength to do was lie on Paula's couch. Vicky would not eat any cake or ice cream but tried to drink some Dr. Pepper. When Vicky got home, I checked her temperature, and it was 100.9. I ground up two Tylenol pills, and put them down Vicky's feed tube. Two hours later Vicky's temperature and heart rate were both lower. Vicky started crying again, and stated that she was sure that she would die if she had to stay in the presence of second hand smoke. Vanessa and I prayed with Vicky, and she calmed down. I helped Vicky wash her mouth, especially in the area of the mouth sore. Vicky cried because of the pain associated with the mouth sore. Vicky was feeling real low and called Sister Sheila for comfort.

At 4:30 Sunday morning, Vicky woke me up. She was crying, and said that she was worried about how she was feeling. Vicky's head would hurt every time her blood pressure went low or high. The pain would pulse with her heart rate. When blood counts were low her heart rate would go up, and her head really hurt badly. I checked her temperature, and it was 101. I ground up two Tylenol to put down the feed tube. I prayed, and laid my head on Vicky's bed until she went back to sleep. I was convinced that I could continue to give Tylenol, and not go to the emergency room, as long as Vicky's temperature would go back down. I couldn't have been more wrong.

Vicky did not want to get out of bed Sunday morning. Vanessa started a home cooked meal while I got Windle and Stacy ready for church. This was the first home cooked meal prepared for the family in many weeks because of Vicky's complications. When I returned from church, Vicky's temperature was 102. I finally realized that Vicky's temperature was not staying down. I called the hospital, and the oncologist told me to take Vicky to the emergency room. The family ate in shifts as Vanessa and I packed for the trip to Children's Hospital. Stacy and Windle were dropped off at Wal Mart to stay with Terry when he got off work.

When Vicky arrived at the emergency room, her blood pressure was low, her heart rate was high, and her temperature was elevated. Vicky's weight was 114 pounds. Blood cultures were obtained, and one liter of fluid was pushed over one hour in her IV. Antibiotics were started, and the doctors started looking for the source of the infection. Blood pressure was monitored closely in case the port was infected; however, her blood pressure remained stable. The blood test showed that Vicky's platelet level was very low, and two units of platelets were transfused.

I used all of the notes, graphs, and history on Vicky to prevent a trip to intensive care. The emergency room doctors were primarily concerned about a possible infection in Vicky's port. If it were infected, the introduction of antibiotics would create a shower of toxins into her blood stream. A shower of toxins would put Vicky in a sepsis condition where her blood pressure would rapidly drop. Vanessa and I started to pray for healing. Vicky's blood pressure remained stable, and she was transferred to the oncology ward on 3 Gold. An additional liter of fluids was required to return blood pressure to normal, and reduce the heart rate to normal. Vicky's head finally stopped hurting. Doctor Stine rightfully counseled me for not bringing Vicky in when her fever first showed up. The fever was eating up platelets, and the blood vessels were slowly dilating. If I had stayed home and gave Tylenol again, Vicky might not have lived. Doctor Stine reminded me that a fever is the first indication of trouble. If you wait until blood pressure drops, and heart rate increases, the child's health can change almost instantly.

By Monday morning Vicky's blood pressure and heart rate had returned to normal, but she continued to spike a fever. The blood cultures were negative for any type of infection in the blood. I went home Monday night to take care of the kids, and Vanessa stayed with Vicky.

On Tuesday, Vicky's blood test showed that she needed two units of red blood. When the doctors made their rounds in the morning, Vicky asked for her feed tube to be removed. The pediatrician agreed to remove the feed tube if Vicky would eat at least five bites of a sandwich. Vicky complied, and the feed tube was removed. After one hour, the nurse reported that Vicky had not touched any more food, and the feed tube was put back in. Vicky was disappointed and depressed, but the feed tube was the only way Vicky could get her pills down.

On Thursday, November 13, Vicky needed two units of platelets. Liquid feeds were started at 50 milliliters per hour, which was one-third the normal rate. The rate of liquid feeds was started at a low rate to ensure that Vicky's intestinal tract would tolerate the feeds. I drove to the hospital after work to stay the night with Vicky and Vanessa. Vanessa and I went to town for dinner and a quiet time together. Vicky's doctor informed her that it would take at least five more days before she could go home. Vicky was looking at her calendar, and noticed that her next round of chemotherapy was scheduled at the same time as her Christmas Party. Vicky asked Doctor Stine if her next round of chemotherapy could be delayed a week so that she could go to the Arkansas Children's Dreams Christmas Party. Doctor Stine was sure that Vicky would not be ready for the next round of chemotherapy before the Christmas Party. I drove back to work early Friday morning and then back home after work.

On Friday, Vicky needed two more units of red blood and one more unit of platelets. During the day, Vanessa and Vicky worked on crafts and puzzles. I looked at my record of Vicky's blood counts. I noticed that between August 1 and November 15, Vicky received 23 units of red blood and 15 units of platelets.

After helping one of the ladies of the church move Saturday; I brought Windle and Stacy to the hospital to visit with Vicky. Vicky was hungry and wanted Taco Bell beans with cheese. When I returned from Taco Bell, Vicky removed her own feed tube without asking the doctor and started eating. Blood test results indicated that Vicky's phosphorus level was low. Vicky refused to take the liquid form of phosphorus she was prescribed now that her feed tube was removed. Her pediatrician found a pill form with phosphorus in it. Vicky had to take six potassium phosphorus (K-phos) pills each day to maintain an adequate phosphorus level. She was willing to take six more pills to keep from putting the feed tube back in. Vicky wanted to go to the Teen room on the fourth floor to play games with other kids her own age. Vicky's white count was still too low to remove her from protective isolation, so Vicky had to stay in her room. Vicky was feeling so good she wanted to stay alone with her nurses. Barbara was going to give Vicky a bath and rub her down with lotion from Victoria's Secret. Vicky reminded me that I was not allowed to put lotion on her feet. Vanessa, Windle, Stacy, and I went to a motel for the night.

During the night one of Vicky's I.V. pumps alarmed. Vicky pushed the call button and told the nurse about the alarm. When Vicky needed to use the bathroom, the pump was still in alarm, so Vicky pushed the emergency call button. Three nurses immediately came running into Vicky's room. Vicky thought it was pretty funny. While the nurses where there, Vicky asked her nurse to pop a bag of cheese popcorn. Vicky ate it all, and later asked for another bag to be popped. I took Windle and Stacy back home Sunday night, and Vanessa stayed with Vicky.

I arrived at the hospital at 7:30 Monday morning to speak with all of Vicky's doctors. Vicky was ready to be discharged, and Vanessa already had her dressed. Doctor Cadle was the pediatric medical student working with Vicky during the weekdays. I learned that Doctor Cadle's mom worked in the chemistry department at the nuclear plant where I worked. Doctor Cadle gratefully accepted all the work I put into Vicky's medical history. This made me feel good about keeping detailed records. After Vicky was discharged, she wanted to go shopping, but not at the Wal Mart in Little Rock. On the way home Vicky asked to shop at the Wal Mart in Conway. I constantly encouraged Vicky to go shopping. It gave her a reason to get out, and it forced her to use her arms and legs. Most of all Vicky's self image improved each time she found pretty shorts, skirts, or a dress.

Vicky's schoolteacher, Mr. Haltom, came to the house Tuesday afternoon to help with her homework. He brought forms to order graduation materials. Vicky tried on Terry's cap and gown, but they were too big. Vicky's order came to $150.00. She was excited about graduating from high school with her friends.

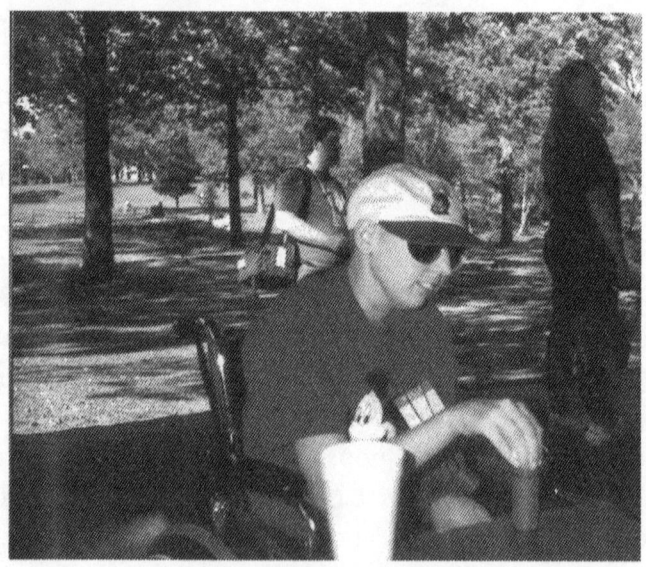

Vicky slowly takes her pills.

THE TRADITION OF THANKSGIVING

Vicky and Vanessa were scheduled to ride the Children's Medical Service (CMS) van to Little Rock on Wednesday, November 20, for a visit to the oncology clinic. The van driver was sick, so I took Vicky while Vanessa stayed at home with Stacy. Vicky had blood work collected the day before by the home health nurse, and the graphs I kept showed that Vicky's platelet count was still dropping 19 days after her last round of chemotherapy. The blood counts obtained at the clinic Wednesday showed the platelet level increasing, but the white blood count was still dropping. I was concerned that there might be an infection brewing which could start eating up platelets. I asked to have two units of platelets transfused since Vicky's platelet level was relatively low. The doctor agreed to the transfusion. When the nurse was transfusing the platelets, she informed me that the more often platelets are given, the more the body rejects them.

I now had something else to consider when monitoring blood counts. Was the slow return of platelets a result of chemotherapy, or radiation, or did platelet transfusions lengthen the recovery time? I also learned that the body adjusts to low platelet counts over time. The nurse said that it was normal to accept low platelet counts and wait as long as possible to see if the body would recover on its own. Rather than looking at graphs alone, I had to accept low platelet counts, and start watching for the signs of very low platelet counts. Bruising around injection sites, and bleeding from the nose or mouth were primary indicators that platelets needed to be transfused. I still relied on my graphs to know when to aggressively look for these signs.

Vicky's appetite had settled on sliced Velveeta cheese and Gatorade. Vicky called me at work Thursday, and asked me to buy some sliced Velveeta cheese on the way home. When I got home, I found out that Vicky had also asked the pastor to pick up some sliced Velveeta cheese and Gatorade. Vicky found it very amusing that it took the pastor over an hour to find the specific cheese she wanted since the pastor does not normally do the grocery shopping. The pastor told Vicky that it would be nice if all members of the church would let others know exactly what they needed.

On Saturday there was a surprise birthday party for Aunt Eunice. Vicky wanted to visit Aunt Eunice, but many of the family members were afraid that Vicky would get sick just by being around so many people. I let Vicky go as long as she promised to wear her mask. Vicky had a wonderful time visiting with all of the women at the party. She stayed for three hours and never once removed her mask. After the party Vicky asked to go shopping with Vanessa at Wal-Mart. I had a board meeting at the church, and I asked Vanessa to give Vicky her injection before going to bed. Vanessa did not want to give the injection, so I woke Vicky up for her shot after I got home from church.

I looked at the chemotherapy schedule with Vicky. There was a good possibility that Vicky would not be able to go to the Christmas church service because of low blood counts or an infection. Vicky made the decision to wear her Christmas outfit Sunday, November 24. She was beautiful in her vest and purple hat she bought at J.C. Penny. Vicky wore her mask to church, and sat with her friend Marcie. After church, Vicky asked to go to Mazzio's where she ate a large cheese lasagna. After eating all of her meal, Vicky ordered and ate another cheese lasagna. Vicky was so excited that her appetite had returned. On the way home from lunch, Vicky had me stop at the grocery store to buy the ingredients for cheese enchiladas. While Vanessa and Vicky took a nap, I made cheese enchiladas. Vicky ate a cheese enchilada before going to the evening church service. After the evening service, Vicky stopped at Taco Bell, and ate a taco salad. Vanessa and I were impressed with Vicky's appetite.

Vanessa and Windle had appointments with their doctors in Fort Smith on Monday. Windle was on a drug study for his epilepsy. Windle also had tourette syndrome and attention deficit disorder (ADD). This new medication was helping to control all three conditions. Windle did not have to go back to his doctor until March of next year. Vanessa's appointment found several problems. Vanessa was scheduled for a technecium heart study and a sleep apnea study. Vanessa was prescribed an antibiotic for an infection and another medication for arthritis pain in her legs and hips. Vicky was hungry, and asked to eat lunch in Fort Smith. She ate two helpings of macaroni and cheese before going back home.

During the drive home from Fort Smith, Vanessa and Vicky talked about setting the house up for Thanksgiving and Christmas. Vanessa was hosting the Thanksgiving meal for several families this year. Vicky was excited about the upcoming holidays. Vanessa's sister normally had the Thanksgiving meal at her house, but she died of cancer. Uncle Phillip and Uncle Marvin were expecting Vanessa to pick up Aunt Sheila's responsibility. After picking up Vanessa's prescriptions and shopping at Wal-Mart, Vicky asked to eat dinner at Mazzio's. Vicky ate two orders of cheese lasagna for dinner again.

Vanessa lay down after getting home because of a severe headache. I put the piano on the front porch to make room for the holidays just like Vicky and Vanessa talked about on the way home. When Vanessa woke up, she noticed what I had done. Vanessa started screaming violently and demanded that everything be put back the way it was. Part of what Vanessa wanted back was her sister. Vanessa went back to bed in a fit of rage. Vicky started crying because she believed that Vanessa hated her for having cancer. Every idea that Vicky had for the holidays was rejected in Vanessa's fit of rage. Vicky was getting so upset that she was having trouble breathing.

I called the pastor and spoke about all of the issues facing Vanessa and her reactions to them. I checked on Vicky after talking with the pastor. She was so upset she wanted to die. I called the pastor back and asked to bring Vicky over for counseling. Vicky started to calm down as she got dressed. Sister Sheila, Marcie, and the pastor spoke with Vicky for over an hour. They addressed Vanessa's health, Vanessa's loss of her sister, and the many issues cancer brought into our family. Vicky and I went home feeling much better, and found Vanessa in a very good mood. Vanessa and I were up until midnight arranging the house for the holidays. The piano stayed on the porch.

Vicky called me at work Tuesday and asked me to bring home cheese lasagna, pizza, and Gatorade for dinner. When I got home, I found the living room beautifully arranged for the holidays. When I tucked Vicky into bed, she demanded that Vanessa come and give her a hug. Vicky called Mom back for another hug shortly after the first one. After Vanessa went back to bed, she asked me to get her evening medications because her legs hurt too much to get back up. I noticed that half of Vanessa's medications for the day was skipped. Vanessa's hips and knees started hurting so badly that she asked me for two additional pain pills. Vanessa said that cleaning house made her legs hurt this badly. Twice during the night Vicky asked for a glass of Gatorade. I got up because Vanessa couldn't get up on her legs.

Vanessa taught Vicky how to make the dressing for the turkey Wednesday evening. Vicky was having so much fun being involved in the preparation of the Thanksgiving meal. Vicky wished that Aunt Sheila were there to help. Vicky was doing a good job of using her left arm for several hours. Vicky was amazed to learn what all went into the dressing and what wasn't in the dressing. Vicky then cut up fruit and made the fruit salad. Everyone started talking about what a great time this was when I reminded everyone that today was the one-year anniversary of Vicky's diagnosis. There really was a lot to be thankful for!

On Thanksgiving day Uncle Phillip and Uncle Marvin came over for lunch. Vicky reminded everyone of who made the dressing, and what was in it. She tried to get Windle to eat dressing by telling him what was not in it. Of course Vicky did not eat any of the dressing, but she did eat Uncle Marvin's macaroni and cheese. Uncle Phillip and Uncle Marvin left when Uncle Marvin started to complain of a headache. I went to Aunt Donna's and brought home a piece of coconut pie for Vicky. Vicky put together a meal for me to take to a family in the church that Terry and I had recently moved. After the evening sunset, the family put up the Christmas tree. Each of the kids placed their personal decoration on the tree they received on their first birthdays. Terry had several packages already wrapped to put under the tree. There was such a wonderful feeling in the night air! Vicky had hugs and kisses for everyone.

On Friday the home health nurse came to the house for Vicky's blood work. I called children's hospital for the results, and I was told to stop the injections to increase the white blood count after Monday night. The platelet count was still low, and Vicky's red blood count was still dropping. I added the values to my graphs. Vicky called me and asked me to bring home some Gatorade. When I got home, Vicky and Vanessa wanted to eat dinner at Pizza Hut. Vicky ate three slices of pepperoni pizza with black olives.

Vicky went to town with me Saturday to find a Christmas gift for Kara. On the way back home Vicky asked to eat at a Mexican restaurant. She ate cheese dip and a taco salad. Vicky and I spent the time at lunch talking about what Vicky wanted to do when she graduated from high school. Vicky spent the afternoon with Vanessa wrapping Christmas gifts. Vanessa and Vicky talked about Mom and Aunt Sheila growing up. Vicky asked Mom if the two of them could sleep together. Vicky was missing Aunt Sheila. I slept in Vicky's bed looking at the many stuffed animals Vicky received at the hospital. Little things like a toy rally can make you feel better. I hugged a big white teddy bear and went to sleep.

Vicky was excited about going to church Sunday morning. She stood at the door with the pastor to greet everyone. Vicky smiled when one family did all they could to get away from her. Vicky took the liberty to invite the pastor, his wife, and Marcie to Mazzio's for pizza. Of course Brother Dade could eat spaghetti. Vicky said that it was to celebrate Mom and Dad's 24th wedding anniversary. Vanessa and Vicky stayed home with Windle and Stacy while I went to the evening church service. Terry was still at work when I got home.

The home health nurse came out for Vicky's blood work Monday morning. Vicky paged me several times during the day. First she wanted to go out for tacos, and I would not agree. She then called back asking me to pick up the ingredients to make tacos at home. The last time Vicky paged me, she wanted permission to give herself her last injection. Vicky grated the cheese while I fixed the rest of the dinner.

Vicky went with Vanessa and I to Fort Smith for Vanessa's technecium heart study Tuesday. Vicky asked to go shopping while Vanessa was taking her test. For lunch Vicky asked to eat at a Mexican restaurant. She did not eat very much of her lunch. I called to check on Vicky's blood counts after lunch, and the platelet count was not high enough to start chemotherapy. Vicky's red blood count was very low. She was scheduled for a direct admission to Children's hospital for two units of red blood on Friday. Vanessa went back to Fort Smith Wednesday to finish up her heart study. Vicky was very tired, and did not want to do anything during Vanessa's test. Vanessa and Vicky packed their bags Thursday. Vicky and Vanessa asked to take a vacation in Little Rock over the weekend.

On Friday, December 6, Vicky was admitted to children's hospital at 8:30 a.m. for two units of red blood. Both clinic 3 and day medicine were full, which required Vicky to be direct admitted for observation on the 3 Gold ward. Carol Godfrey asked me to bring Vicky in for chemotherapy on Tuesday instead of Monday because of so many admissions already scheduled for Monday.

Vanessa and I used a two-for-one coupon to stay Friday and Saturday night at one of the downtown motels. Vanessa, Stacy, and Windle went to the motel while I stayed with Vicky. Jenny Brown, with channel 11 news, was doing interviews with kids at Children's Hospital for a Christmas special. Vicky was asked if she would like to be interviewed, and she was pleased to do so. After the interview, I gave Jenny a copy of Vicky's booklet to become more familiar with Vicky.

I spoke with doctor Stine about predicting Vicky's blood counts from the graphs I was creating. Doctor Stine was satisfied with requesting a transfusion of platelets when they fell below 10. He was also satisfied with scheduling day medicine when blood counts were anticipated to be at a transfusion level. However, doctor Stine would not agree to going to the emergency room on a weekend if counts were low, unless there was a medical need. There would have to be active bleeding, difficulty breathing, or other such physical signs of low blood counts.

After leaving the hospital Friday night at 10:00 p.m., Vicky asked to go to Mazzio's for some cheese lasagna. Vicky ate lasagna until Mazzio's closed. Vicky and I arrived at the motel near midnight.

Vicky asked to eat from the breakfast buffet at the motel in the morning. The family then went to one of the malls downtown where Vicky looked in every store. After a lunch of pizza, Vicky wanted the family to go to the Robinson Center for a Christmas program. Vicky walked from the parking lot to the auditorium and back. This was almost a one-mile walk. After the Christmas program, the family went back to the motel to watch the Christmas parade. For dinner Vicky asked to eat pizza at Pizza Hut. On the way to dinner, I parked the car to watch the fireworks over the capitol. Then Mickey Mouse turned on one million lights around the capitol. The sight was breath taking. After dinner, Vicky wanted to see the Christmas lights on the Ronald McDonald House before going back to the motel. The lights at the McDonald House were beautiful.

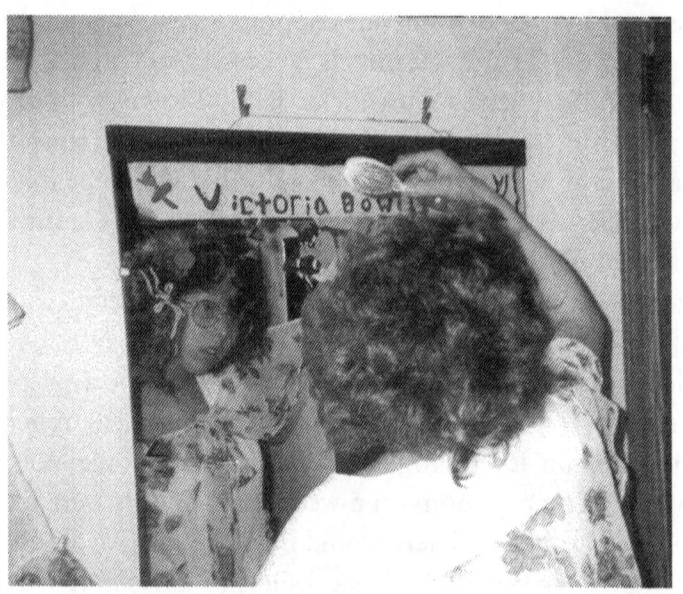

Vicky fixing her wig before company arrived.

THE CHRISTMAS SPIRIT

After breakfast at McDonald's, Vicky asked to tour the Ronald McDonald house. There was a beautiful display in the reading room that Vicky was most impressed with. The hallways were beautifully decorated for Christmas. On one of the chairs in the cancer wing was a quilt Vanessa finished while Vicky was in intensive care. The kids asked to hurry up and go to the Christmas party.

The Children's Dreams Christmas Party was at the Hilton Inn. The first thing each child did was to enter Santa's workshop to select a gift. Vicky wanted a stuffed Bugs Bunny, Windle selected a farm set, and Stacy picked out jewelry. There were sandwiches, pizza, cookies, and all kinds of drinks for everyone. Vanessa and I visited with several families we knew from the intensive care unit, or the McDonald's House. Some of the families were finished with chemotherapy, and had good reports. When Santa arrived, the presentation of gifts started. Both channel 11 and channel 4 were on hand to cover the party, with channel 11 conducting an interview with Vicky.

Santa's helpers called Vicky to sit on Santa's lap. She returned to the table with the telephone she wanted. When Stacy was called, she returned with a box 5 feet tall and 2 feet square. Stacy was dancing with joy as she tore off the wrapping. The channel 11 camera closed in on Stacy as she took the wrapping off her present and found a vanity set. Over one hundred kids were called after Stacy before Windle was called. Windle was getting worried that his name might be missed and asked everyone in the area to listen for his name. When his name was called, Windle jumped up, and ran to Santa's lap in front of another child.

Windle returned with his present and opened it. "A computer!" he shouted. This was a wonderful event to take Vicky, Windle, and Stacy to. Stacy's vanity set barely fit into the car.

On the way home Vicky asked to stop at Mazzio's for cheese lasagna again. Stacy fell asleep on the floor as Windle and Vicky rehearsed the day's events. Once the family was home, Vicky made me change out the phone. Stacy woke up to play with her vanity, and Windle played with his computer until 10:00 at night. There was a beautiful Christmas spirit in the air.

I had to obtain a letter from Vicky's pediatrician in Russellville transferring her to the care of the oncology department at Children's hospital in order to obtain Department of Human Services (DHS) assistance. In the event the CMS van could not take Vicky to an appointment in Little Rock, DHS would pay mileage expenses. But, the request must be made before the trip occured, and CMS transportation had to be unavailable. Payment would not be allowed for a trip to the hospital if a request for mileage did not occur before the trip. In order to get round trip mileage the hospital had to fax a statement of intent to release or discharge to DHS before the return trip mileage could be applied for. I was amazed at all of the government red tape.

On December 10, I drove Vanessa and Vicky to Little Rock to start the next round of chemotherapy. I stopped at a Total gas station in Conway for Vicky to go to the bathroom. There was a woman in the store with short black hair and several earrings in her left ear. She had on a white Mickey Mouse sweat shirt and faded blue jeans. As Vanessa left the store, the woman asked if Vicky liked Winnie the Pooh, and Vanessa said yes. When Vicky and I came out of the store, the woman presented Vicky with a Winnie the Pooh stuffed animal, and said "Merry Christmas." The woman then went to the front of the store. As I drove away, Vanessa and Vicky looked for the woman to thank her, but she was nowhere to be seen. Was she an angel? Vicky wanted to think so.

After Vicky was admitted to the hospital, she sent me out to Mazzio's for pizza. Vicky ate 5 slices of pepperoni pizza for lunch. Some of Vicky's friends from school were visiting the hospital, and they gave Vicky two stuffed animals. Vicky was glad to see some of her school friends. The doctors and nurses from the clinic also gave Vicky a teddy bear. Vicky curled up to all five of her stuffed animals; Pooh, Bugs, and three teddy bears. Janet was Vicky's nurse, and Vicky was having fun being "Sassy."

Janet was Vicky's nurse for all three days of chemotherapy. On Wednesday Doctor Nicholas ordered an X-ray of Vicky's left arm, and noted that everything looked good. Janet woke Vicky up Thursday morning by shinning a flashlight into her eyes at 6:30 in the morning. Vicky was extra "Sassy" with Janet for the rude awakening. Vicky was released Thursday morning just before lunch. On the way home Vicky stopped at the American Cancer Society to look at wigs. Vicky picked out a beautiful red wig that reminded her of Reba McEntire.

At home Vicky begged me to take her to see the movie "101 Dalmatians." Vicky, Terry, and I went to see the movie. While there Vicky ate popcorn and took all of her pills. On the way home Vicky asked to eat at a Mexican restaurant. She ate a few bites of a cheese enchilada. There was a person in the restaurant smoking, and Vicky started having trouble breathing, and her appetite went away. When we got home, Terry showed Mom three lumps in the muscle of his right fore arm. The thought of cancer in another child was more than Vanessa could take. Vanessa called Sister Sheila and asked her to pray for the family. Vicky had the sniffles and asked for a Benadryl at bedtime.

On the 13th Terry went to see his pediatrician about the lumps in his arm. With Vicky having cancer, we did not want to take any chances. The doctor agreed and made an appointment with a dermatologist. Vicky paged me at work, and asked me to bring home Spanish rice, orange coke, and cream cheese. We spent the evening working on Christmas cards. Vanessa and I questioned if this would be a good

Christmas if Terry had cancer. We tried to put the thought out of our minds, but Vicky's medical supplies were a constant reminder.

On Saturday, December 14, Vanessa, Stacy, and Windle went to a Christmas party for kids where the movie "101 Dalmatians" was showing. Vicky took me shopping at the mall while the move was showing. When we all got home, Vicky, Stacy, and Windle worked together to make a birthday cake for Terry. We celebrated Terry's birthday when he got home from work. On Sunday Vicky wanted to go to church even though her counts were low. Vicky sat in the back of the Church for Sunday school and the main service because of her white blood count being low. Limiting the number of people Vicky came in contact with reduced the chances of her getting an infection from other people. After church, Vicky finished the Christmas cards.

Home health come to the house Monday morning, and the results of the blood test showed a need for blood and platelets during the week. The Phenobarbital level was now at a proper therapeutic level. Vanessa went to Windle's school for his play, but it was canceled because the former principle died of cancer. The school was closed the next day for the funeral. Vicky paged me at work, and asked me to bring home cheese lasagna from Mazzio's. Vicky ate half of the lasagna. On Tuesday Vicky gave her own injection without any numbing cream, and she did fine. Vicky asked to take more control of her medications.

Vicky made cup cakes for me to take to church Wednesday night. She received a package from Reba McEntire's office with a card and cassette tape. The family listened to Reba all day long. Vicky wanted to try giving her injection into her left arm. A small bruise, called teaki eye, appeared at the injection site. Vicky's platelet level was obviously low. It was time to watch for signs of bleeding.

Home health came out Thursday to draw blood again. The red blood count was 5.0, and platelets were 2.0. The blood counts were very low. Vicky lay in bed all day long because of a lack of energy. When I got home from work, Vicky had blood in her mouth, and she was bleeding from her nose. Vicky started crying, and stated that she was scared of how she was feeling. I called the hospital, and headed for the emergency room at Children's Hospital. Vicky was admitted to the hospital for transfusions.

On Friday Vicky was transfused with two units of platelets and three units of red blood. Vanessa and I met the parents of a 13-year-old girl just diagnosed with leukemia. Kara was still in the hospital with a fever from an infection. During the day Vicky did not eat anything, and her mouth was coated white with thrush. Vicky was discharged at 6:30 p.m. On the way home, Vicky bought some candy and ice cream, and ate a few bites. When Vicky arrived at home, she found a basket of fruit sent by grandma and grandpa. Vicky spent hours on the phone talking with grandpa, her Uncle Marvin, and her Cousin Paula.

Saturday Vicky started taking mouth care seriously. She was scrubbing her tongue with nystatin and the hemoc mouthwash. The thrush was in check, and Vicky's mouth was free of mouth sores. Vicky sent me to town for a chocolate donut. Every time Vicky had a bowel movement she cried because of pain, and there was a small amount of blood. Vicky called the pastor's wife for permission to attend church the next day because of the white count being so low. Sister Sheila told Vicky to wear her mask and stay away from crowds.

Vicky and Vanessa spent days making several Christmas gifts for Vicky's friends and teachers at church. Vicky also went out and purchased a few other presents. Vicky took a bag full of presents to church with her. Vicky passed out presents in the morning, and then went to her Sunday school class where she shared a tin of chocolates with her classmates. Vicky slid the chocolates under her mask and the mask was covered with traces of candy. The children's church performed a beautiful Christmas Program in the morning service. Vicky was glad she was able to see the program. Vicky was excited when she was handed a bag of treats from the church when she left at the end of the service. Vicky was more excited about Christmas this year than ever.

Between the morning and evening service, Vicky cleaned out all of her dresser drawers. I baked a blackberry pie for the fellowship meal at the church. Vicky could hardly wait to eat and fellowship at church after the evening service.

Vicky wore her new red wig to the evening service, and everyone raved about it. Communion was served following the evening service, and Vicky participated. Vicky believed that the communion service was instrumental in her feeling so good. At the evening meal, Vicky ate mashed potatoes and baked beans—lots of them! Vicky had a wonderful time of fellowship with everyone during the meal. Several families sent food home with Vicky when the meal was all over.

On Monday morning Vicky woke me up by squirting me with a 20-cc syringe full of ice cold water. She demanded that I take her to the donut shop for breakfast. Vicky called home health, and told them that she would see them at the office. Vicky had no intention of staying around the house.

For breakfast Vicky ate a chocolate donut and biscuits with gravy. At the home health office, Vicky met, and played with, Amanda Morrow's newborn child. Vicky's white blood count was 4.5 so she no longer needed her mask. Vicky attributed the quick return of her white count to communion and prayer. Carol Godfrey suggesting that Vicky take her white count to 10.0 with injections may have played a role in rapid recovery. But, in six days Vicky's white count recovered, which was a record. Vicky was positive God healed her. She expected God to do the same for the lumps in Terry's arm.

Vicky had two shopping lists with her at the grocery store. One was for the Christmas Eve meal at home, and the other was for the Christmas meal at Aunt Paula's home. Vicky planned on eating, and eating, and eating again. Vicky and I went to several grocery stores to get all of the items on the two lists.

When Vicky got back home she made cookies and arranged snack trays for the two Christmas parties. Vicky cleaned her bedroom, vacuumed the house, cleaned Windle's room, and cleaned her bathroom in preparation for the Christmas eve party at the house. Vicky then walked to Aunt Eunice's and visited for a long time. The excitement of Christmas was all over Vicky.

On Christmas Eve, Vicky made her Christmas dip that everyone enjoyed. Vicky went over to Paula's and spent several hours with her preparing for the Christmas meal. Vicky snacked on chips and dip all day long. Just before going to bed, Stacy, Windle, and Vicky opened their presents from Aunt Shirley and one additional present. Windle was so excited that his tourette syndrome tics were showing up very much. It took a long time for all of the kids to fall asleep. Santa went to work.

Vicky was the first one up Christmas morning at 4:30. She claimed to be hungry, and wanted me to get her some chips and dip. Finally at 5:15, Vicky had all she could stand, and woke everyone up. She had not touched any of her food. Vicky found a Taz pillow wearing a pair of Taz panties, and plenty of toys. After all was cleaned up, the family opened the wrapped presents under the tree. Vicky's favorite gift was a Mickey designer short suit, which she wore all day. Terry surprised me with a Mosberg 12-gauge pump shotgun. Presents for other family members were packed into Terry's truck, and everyone followed him over to Paula's house. Uncle Marvin was there, and he was totally paralyzed in the left arm and leg. The headache he had on Thanksgiving Day was a stroke. It was good to have him with the family.

Paula served sandwiches and snacks for lunch, and Vicky ate chips, dip, and sweet pickles. Presents flowed like water for a good while with so many people present. After spending four hours with Paula, Vicky wanted to go back home. Vicky helped Windle put his wood models together before she went to bed.

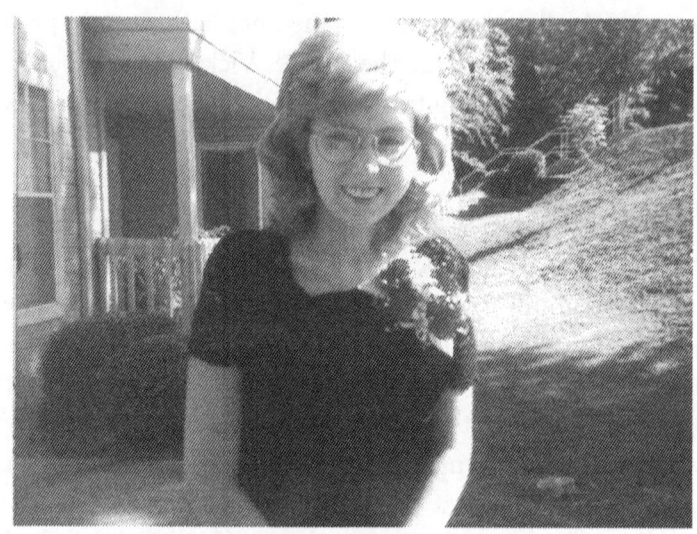

Vicky dressed for church.

THE STRESS OF IT ALL

Mary, the home health nurse, woke Vicky up for her blood test Thursday, December 26. Vicky noticed me getting ready to go to work, and asked if she could go with me. Vicky quickly dressed and went to work with me. Vicky used a computer for four hours typing letters to her friends. The longer she worked, the more she used her left hand on the keyboard. Vicky and I talked about what to have for dinner, and Vicky wanted to go to Dixie Cafe in Fort Smith using a gift certificate I won in a safety meeting.

At the Dixie Cafe, Vicky ate a little of her applesauce and ice cream, and boxed the rest to take home. When the family got back home, Terry showed the movie "Independence Day." Vicky stayed up until 2:30 in the morning watching the movie, and visiting with Terry.

Friday morning Vanessa and I went to buy groceries, and had the oil changed in the Ford Tempo. When we got home, the water to the house was turned off. I had to pay $160.00 to have the water service restored which left no money to buy Vicky's and Vanessa's medications for the next two weeks. The family had to relocate to Little Rock in two weeks for Vicky's radiation treatments, and I was stressed with all of the finances. I had borrowed money to have Christmas, and I borrowed money to make the house payments.

Many people provided money at the beginning of Vicky's illness, and others were supporting the family on a monthly basis. During the first round of radiation with relocation to Little Rock, I had to use all of the family savings. The out-of-pocket expenses for the first year of Vicky's illness averaged $500.00 per month. Now at the end of 1996, all of the family finances were exhausted, and I didn't know where to go next. The financial stress pushed Vanessa beyond her ability to cope, and I was close to that same point.

I felt the leading of the Spirit to go and see Dr. Jack Glaze at New Life Academy in Clarksville. Dr. Glaze gave me the money needed to make the next house payment. When I got back home, the water was turned on. Until you have a family member with a serious illness, like cancer, you don't realize the heavy financial burden placed on the family. During the next two weeks, friends at my work provided financial gifts that met every need. Vicky said, "God uses people to take care of all the needs."

During the time that I was meeting with Dr. Glaze, Vanessa was quilting a blanket. Stacy and Windle were making a mess of the house, and Vicky was in bed. Vicky's medications were two hours late, and she did not have anything to eat or drink all morning. When I pressed Vanessa to help with all that needed to be done, she reacted to the stress by going to bed. I got Vicky's medications down, and tried to get her to eat. Vicky asked for some chicken noodles, and I made them. Vicky ate two bites, and went back to bed. I was begging Vicky to eat something when Vanessa woke up. Vanessa suggested Mazzio pizza to Vicky, and I tried to talk them out of going because of the cost. But, Vicky and Vanessa were set on going to Mazzio's Pizza. Vicky was moving slowly as if her blood counts were really low.

At Mazzio's, Vicky ordered lasagna and a salad bar, and I used coupons to keep the cost as low as possible. Vicky barely ate her food and asked for a to-go box. When the family got back home, Vanessa went back to bed. I gave Vicky her evening pills, her injection and did her mouth care. While doing Vicky's mouth care, she became nauseated, and gave up all of her dinner. I gave her medication for the nausea. I wanted so desperately to run away. I now fully understood what Gregg Adams meant about families with cancer. He said that half of the married families who have kids with cancer divorce. The stresses were the root cause. I prayed and asked God for strength.

Shawnee, Vicky's cousin, called to tell Vicky that Karen Wheaton would be at the Conway High School on January 17. I cleaned the living room, and was working on the kitchen when Vicky said she was hungry. Vicky ate half of a grilled cheese sandwich, drank a grape drink, and had two sweet pickles for dessert. Finally at 10:30, Vicky asked for lights out and all of her Taz animals and pillows. The thought of seeing Karen Wheaton sparked a hope in Vicky.

On Saturday, December 28, Vicky woke up Mom, and asked if the two could go to the Dollar Store. Vicky bought some flowers, and placed them on Aunt Sheila's grave. Terry and I went under the house to insulate the ductwork, and lay plastic on the ground under the house. Vicky asked me to go out with her to rake leaves. I mulched with the lawn mower while Vicky racked. Vicky talked about seeing Karen Wheaton soon.

Paula brought her mom's (aunt Sheila) clothes over to the house for Vicky to try on. Vicky was able to fit into so many of the clothes. Vicky walked up to Aunt Eunice's house to visit while Vanessa and Stacy took a nap. Vicky took some of the cloths over to Johnna Boone. Vanessa insisted on eating a hamburger in town, and Vicky wanted to go to the Diamond Drive Inn. Vicky met three of her classmates at the restaurant. Vicky and her classmates talked about the prom. Vicky ate two bites of her cheeseburger; half of her french fries, and half of a chocolate ice cream cone. Vicky did her own mouth care before going to bed.

Vicky put on her new blue dress she got for Christmas Sunday morning. Vicky made the dress look beautiful. After church Johnna Boone took Vicky to Wendy's for lunch. Vanessa complained of her right knee hurting badly. After lunch, Vanessa went to bed. Vicky called Aunt Eunice for a taco casserole recipe. Vicky and Vanessa cooked taco casserole for dinner while I was at the evening church service.

Vicky got up Monday morning when the home health nurse arrived. Vicky wanted the family to get dressed so she could eat biscuits and gravy at the donut shop. At the donut shop, Vicky was trying to take the bandage off of her arm where the nurse took blood. Vanessa reached over, and pulled the bandage quickly. Vicky's arm immediately bruised because of a low platelet count. Vicky got mad that Mom bruised her. It was time once again to look for signs of bleeding. Vicky went shopping at Wal Mart, and bought one of the "Christi" videos. Back at the house, Vicky stuffed envelopes with her Christmas letter she typed at my work.

Vanessa's leg was hurting much more Tuesday, and she took a nap right after lunch. Vicky took the time to clean her room. For dinner Vicky ate two grilled cheese sandwiches and a bowl of chicken noodle soup.

On the last day of the year, Vicky called me at work to meet me for lunch. I took the family to Arby's, and Vicky ate a few french fries. Terry and I spent the afternoon working on his truck. The three lumps in Terry's arm looked much larger. Sister Sheila arrived to visit with Vicky, and Vicky didn't want her to leave. All Vicky could eat for dinner was a grilled cheese sandwich. Vanessa asked me to make an appointment to have her knee checked.

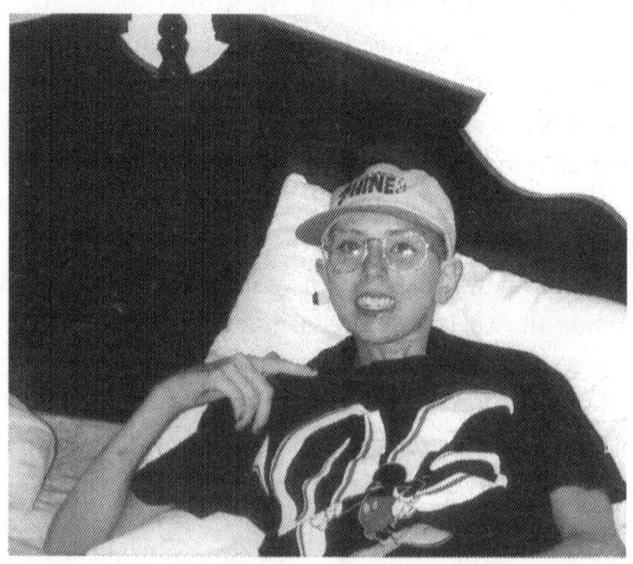

Vicky modeling her hat from David Ring. It says "Don't whine, SHINE."

LET'S GO SEE KAREN

The first day of 1997 started out with a lazy morning for Vicky. She decided to stay in bed until noon. Terry and I spent part of the morning working on his truck. I then installed a set of low voltage lights in the garden I bought over two years ago. Vicky was in the mood to go visiting after getting out of bed. She called Ray and Zetta, but they already had plans for the day. Vicky then asked me if the family could go to Cline Park for a picnic.

It was a warm 68 degrees at the park, and the air was still. Vicky asked to cook hot-dogs on the grill. Watching Vicky and Stacy swing while smelling hot dogs cook made me think back to days when Vicky was Stacy's age. Life was much easier then. Vicky ate a hot dog, sweet pickles, and Cheetos. The family then spent the afternoon playing on the swings. Vicky was having so much fun swinging with Stacy. The family stayed at the park until the sun went down and the cool night air set in. Vanessa said that her right knee was hurting all the time now. When the pastor returned from vacation, I called to let him know about obtaining financial assistance for the water bill and house payment. For dinner, Vicky ate cheese popcorn and sweet pickles.

A home health nurse came to the house Thursday morning for Vicky's blood tests. I asked Vicky what she wanted for breakfast, but she did not want to eat anything. Vicky asked if I would take her to town for breakfast. I told Vicky that I would take her to lunch if she would eat something for breakfast. Vicky ate a few sweet pickles. She then asked to go to Taco Bell for a hard shell taco. When Vicky ate the taco, she immediately got sick to her stomach and headed for the rest room. Nearly twenty minutes passed before Vicky returned. She tried cleaning herself off, and wanted to go home immediately. When I took Vicky back to the house, I called the hospital to check on her blood counts. Her red blood count was low, and she was scheduled for a transfusion at Children's Hospital Friday. I took Vanessa to the hospital in Fort Smith for her sleep study while Terry watched the kids. Everyone was asleep when I got back home.

I picked Vanessa up in Fort Smith early Friday morning. The test results showed that Vanessa does not have sleep apnea, but she does have trouble getting to sleep. Vanessa and I stopped by the house to pick up Vicky, and then went to Children's hospital. On the way, Vicky ate half of a McDonald hash brown and half of a candy bar for breakfast. Vicky looked so frail with her head slumped over. I tried to lift Vicky's spirits, but I knew that the low blood counts were controlling the desire to be "Sassy."

At clinic 3, Vanessa and Vicky met and talked with Nan Brooks. Nan's son was in intensive care for the side effects of chemotherapy at the same time Vicky was in intensive care. Vicky was admitted to room 3125 for her blood transfusions. Vicky weighed 109 pounds, and her blood pressure was good. Vicky sent Vanessa and I to the grocery store for foods she wanted to eat during the day.

Vanessa and I returned from grocery shopping with sweet pickles, sliced Velveeta cheese, chicken noodle soup, and roman noodles. Rhonda was Vicky's nurse, and Vicky found out that Rhonda would be a year older on Tuesday. The first unit of red blood was type A (Rh positive), and second unit was type O (Rh positive). I was told that type O blood was universal. Type A blood was not available for the second unit because of the high use of blood and low donations during the holidays.

Doctor Gregg Gilliam, with infectious control, stated that no other patient at Children's hospital had VRE. Good hand washing was instrumental in the control of this form of bacteria. I thought about the fears of people who wanted to throw Vicky out of church. I wondered if they would receive the report, or continue to avoid Vicky. I felt it was best not to tell them. Gregg Adams stopped by to tell us that he would check on the availability of the Open Arms apartment in Little Rock for Vicky's next round of radiation.

On the way home Friday night Vicky wanted to eat at Shoney's in Conway. Vicky enjoyed eating from the food bar. Vicky tried everything on the food bar. After dinner, the waiter told Vanessa and I not to worry about the bill. A gentleman had asked for our ticket. The waiter and store manager had no idea who the man was. Vicky said that it was another one of her angels. During the ride home, Vicky talked about all of her encounters with angels. Vanessa and I realized it was time for us to study the Bible about angels.

Vicky's physical therapists, Larry and Christina, came to the house Saturday to measure Vicky's movements. Vicky's progress was outstanding. She had regained full use of her right arm, and doubled the function of the left arm. Vicky started on strengthening exercises, such as the ability to balance on one foot. With a lot of work, Vicky was expected to have most of her left arm back by the end of the year.

Vicky asked if she could invite Ray and Zetta over for dinner. Vicky gave them a call, but they could not come until late in the evening. Vicky asked if they would come for snacks. Vicky spent the afternoon baking brownies. For dinner Vicky ate pork and beans with Velveeta cheese melted in them. Vicky then decorated and set the table for snacks. Vicky was a great hostess for the evening. She served pizza, brownies, chips with dip, nuts, and coke. Ray and Zetta enjoyed the time of fellowship as did Vicky and the rest of the family.

Vanessa stayed home from church Sunday morning. Her right knee was very painful, and her right foot was numb. Vicky went to Sunday school, and then worked in Children's church. The one family that tried to throw her out of church got irritated that Vicky was in Children's church and stormed out of the church. Vicky knew that VRE could never hurt them. I knew they would not believe the report from

Children's hospital that VRE was fully controlled. For lunch, Vicky ate three grilled cheese sandwiches. Vicky then called Amanda Morrow to see if she would come over to visit.

Amanda came to visit with Vicky Sunday afternoon. Monday started homecoming week at Johnson County Westside High School. The two spent the afternoon talking about the prom and graduation. Vicky then showed Amanda the videotape of her time in the hospital. After listening to Amanda and Vicky talk, I realized that I must balance giving Vicky more freedom while watching for all of the side effects of cancer and treatments. Vicky's desire to be "Sassy" was largely controlled by her red blood count.

A home health nurse woke Vicky up to take her blood Monday morning. Vicky paged me at work, and asked if I would take her to town after work. Vanessa's leg hurt so badly that she could not get out with Vicky. I made Vanessa an appointment with her doctor for Tuesday afternoon. Vicky paged me again, and asked if she could go to Pizza Hut for dinner. For lunch Vicky ate two grilled cheese sandwiches. I called to talk with Karen Wheaton. Karen was looking forward to meeting with Vicky in Conway. Karen's newest newsletter had the story of Vicky in it. I called Carol Godfrey at Children's hospital to check on the results of Vicky's blood counts. Vicky's platelet level was still at 19. Carol would talk with doctor Stine about the schedule for the next round of chemotherapy. Vicky was scheduled for a clinic visit Wednesday. The weather report was calling for four inches of snow Wednesday. Terry had his appointment for the lumps on his arm. They were just fatty deposits, and had nothing to do with cancer. Vanessa and I were glad to get the good report.

For dinner, Vicky ate two slices of pepperoni pizza and four crackers at Pizza Hut. I then took Vicky shopping at Wal Mart. I helped Vicky with her exercises before she went to bed. Vicky pushed out 20 repetitions of each exercise. Vicky then worked on balancing on one foot. For a bedtime snack, Vicky ate half a grilled cheese sandwich and a sweet pickle. Vicky's stomach became nauseated, and she asked for medication to stop the nausea.

Vicky slept in Tuesday morning. For lunch, she had a grilled cheese sandwich and roman noodles. I watched Vicky and Stacy at the doctor's office while Vanessa visited with her doctor. An X-ray and exam showed that Vanessa had osteo arthritis in her knee. Vanessa will start taking an anti-inflammatory medication. When the medication no longer works, then she would need a steroid shot. When the shots no longer work, then surgery would be needed. Mr. Haltom from the school came to the house to work with Vicky on schoolwork. The forms for taking the ACT test in the hospital were completed.

Vanessa, Stacy, Vicky, and I left for Little Rock Wednesday morning at 5:30. It was sleeting by the time Vicky arrived at the Clinic 3 for a checkup of her heart. Vicky was very nervous for this test. The echogram of the heart checked the central line to see if it was covered with blood clots or if it was interfering with a valve function. The test also measured blood flow velocity, the size of the valves, and the size of the chambers.

Vicky's urinalysis and blood tests results were normal. Depending on the results of the next blood test, Vicky would be scheduled for a full set of scans next Tuesday. Chemotherapy would start the following day, and radiation to the hips and left leg would start the following week. Sometime between the 15th and 20th the family would move back into the Open Arms apartment in Little Rock. The interstate had cleared by the time we went home. I wanted to make plans for Vicky's treatments and my work. I was so frustrated that cancer was controlling my schedule instead of me controlling the cancer. It was at this moment that I realized that the entire family had this cancer, not just Vicky.

A home health nurse woke Vicky up for her blood test Thursday morning. There was no school because of snow and ice on the campus. Vicky called me at work, and asked me to bring home some hard cheese (no more Velveeta) roman noodles, and chicken noodle soup. Gregg

Adams called me at work about the use of the Open Arms apartment. Vicky would stay in the Ronald McDonald house the night before her chemotherapy. When she came out of the hospital, the family would move into the Open Arms apartment.

The school bus picked up Windle for school Friday morning, and returned shortly after because of the snow and ice. Doctor Robinson called Vanessa about her sleep test and blood results. Vanessa is part of five percent of the population with sleep disorders who only need sleeping pills. Her trigliceride level was off scale above 1,200. Vanessa started medications for sleep and to lower the trigliceride level. During the night, Vicky had a dream where two angels took Aunt Sheila to heaven. The dream scared Vicky, and she woke me to wipe the tears and hold her hand. I prayed with Vicky and then fell asleep on the floor next to her bed.

Vicky asked to eat breakfast at a restaurant Saturday morning. All Vicky would eat was two cheese sticks. For lunch Vicky ate a cheese sandwich using hard cheese. I called Doctor Jack Glaze to talk about long term financial assistance. The family ate dinner at Tastee Taco with Doctor Jack Glaze and his two daughters.

It was a cold 17 degrees Sunday morning. Vicky wore her long black dress and long coat to church. After Sunday school, Vicky sat in the nursery to lean back in a rocking chair. She listened to the service on the intercom. There was a little boy in the nursery with Vicky.

Vicky asked to eat lunch at Kentucky Fried Chicken after church. Vicky ate one serving of potatoes and gravy. After lunch, Vicky went to Wal Mart, and bought an outfit for Amanda Morrow's baby. At home, Vicky made two copies of a video she produced. The video has scenes of her in intensive care and other areas of the hospital set to music. One copy was for Amanda, and the other was for Johnna Boone. I took Johnna's copy with me to the evening service at church. Terry's truck would not start after he got off work. He called the house, and Vicky paged me at church. I left the evening service to help Terry start his truck. The positive battery post was loose. Johnna called to see if Vicky could go to the youth rally Monday night. I had to let Vicky make the decision. She asked to go, and I insisted that Vicky wear her mask during the entire service. Vicky agreed to wear her mask. The pastor's wife called to inform me that the boy sitting with Vicky in the nursery was sick with flu-like symptoms. I watched closely to see if Vicky would start running a fever.

Mr. Haltom came to the house Monday for home schooling. Johnson County Westside would control Vicky's homework while the family was in Little Rock so that Vicky could graduate with her classmates. Mr. Holtom would leave homework with Terry, and Terry would deliver completed homework to the school. Johnna Boone picked up Vicky for the youth rally, and I packed for the trip to Little Rock in the morning.

Vicky and I left for Little Rock Tuesday morning, January 14, at 5:00. Vicky's port was accessed and the blood test drawn. The first test Vicky was scheduled for was a MRI of the left shoulder. The radioactive substance called technesium-99 was injected in preparation for the bone scan. The next test was a chest CT scan. The bone scan was last. The radiologist saw a change in the upper right arm, and another bone scan of the right arm was performed. Three reference X-rays of the right arm were taken. Vicky asked to leave her port accessed during the night. Vicky and I checked into the Ronald McDonald house after all of the tests. Vicky checked into room 101 and then bought a McDonald's sweatshirt.

Vicky made herself at home in the dinning area, and started work on a puzzle. Vicky did not want to eat lunch in the hospital cafeteria. For lunch, Vicky made Jell-O, a cheese sandwich, and roman noodles in the McDonald house kitchen. Vicky only ate a fourth of the sandwich. Vicky asked to go to bed at 7:00 p.m. At 9:30, she took her evening pills with some Dr. Pepper. Fifteen minutes later, Vicky emptied the contents of her stomach. I forgot to bring the medication for nausea, and Vicky started missing Mom. Throughout the evening Vicky reacted to the thought of chemotherapy with nausea and a loss of appetite. The doctor warned Vanessa and I that this might happen. It is a conditioned emotional response to the negative side effects of chemotherapy. Vicky was questioning why she had cancer. Vicky's side and back stated hurting, and she was cold. I put all of the blankets on Vicky. Vicky asked me to rub the area over her gall bladder and her back. Vicky cried most of the night. The sound of an ice storm broke the sound of Vicky's tears during the night.

The roads and sidewalks between the McDonald house and the hospital were covered with ice Wednesday morning. I took Vicky to Clinic 3 in a wheel chair because of the ice. Vicky took her morning medications with water, but it all came right back up. The nurse took Vicky's blood tests, and then gave her medication for nausea through the port needle. Vicky finally rested, and went to sleep. I called Vanessa, and she said that the interstate was closed because of ice. Vicky woke up, and asked me to go back to the McDonald house to get her Taz pillow and the blanket Aunt Eunice made because she was cold.

Vicky was admitted to the hospital, and the chemotherapy drug cytoxin would run over 24 hours. The chemotherapy drug, adriamycin could no longer be administered because of the toxicity effects on the lungs. Vicky's CT scan of the lung was normal, but I could see where the last round of radiation clipped the left lung. This was the primary reason adriamycin could no longer be administered. The X-rays of the right arm were normal. The increased activity of the right arm on the bone scan was attributed to the increased use of the right arm in all of Vicky's activities. The echogram of the heart was normal. The MRI scan of the shoulder showed the presence of the residual tumor mass, and it had not grown. It was believed to be scar tissue. The hips on the bone scan looked much better than in the previous bone scans. All in all, the test results were very encouraging. Vicky's doctor indicated that if he had these test results when we first came in, she would have been declared cancer free. But these aren't the tests we came in with. The research shows that you must treat this type of cancer with chemotherapy and radiation to kill it out. The calcium level on the blood test was low, and doctor Stine adjusted the calcium level over the next two days. Vicky was admitted to room 3123 and chemotherapy was started. I went to the parent's support meeting, and then went home to pack for the move into the apartment.

Vanessa, Windle, Stacy, and I moved into the Open Arms apartment Thursday, January 16. I went to the hospital to pick up Vicky. Nan Brook was celebrating the end-of-chemo party with her son. Doctor Stine changed Vicky's magnesium medication to a different type of salt to help raise the magnesium level in the blood. Calcium pills were added because of the low value of calcium on the blood test.

After getting Vicky settled into the apartment, the family went to the grocery store. Vicky was very sluggish from the chemotherapy and nausea medication. Vicky ate a few bites for dinner, but she did not want anymore cheese. As the evening hours arrived, Vicky started to perk up. I contacted a national cancer counseling organization, and Vicky would be placed in contact with a patient, or survivor, who was treated for Ewing's Sarcoma. Vicky felt positive about herself knowing that someone would call her soon. I sent out a request for help with Vicky's emotional state. Many people responded to Vicky's situation, and sent her special words of encouragement, and gifts to occupy her time.

The Pulaski County home health nurses came to the apartment Friday, January 17 for their required assessment and blood tests. Vicky was very much awake and gave Kyla a very "Sassy" welcome back. Vicky did not eat any breakfast, and only had half a serving of mashed potatoes from Kentucky Fried Chicken for lunch. Vicky took medication for nausea and a nap before going to see Karen Wheaton in Conway. Carol Godfrey called, and Vicky was scheduled for a blood transfusion Tuesday in the day medicine clinic. I gave Vicky her injection before leaving for the concert. Vicky put on her blue Christmas dress, her red wig, and a necklace made of letters that reads: "LET'S GO SEE KAREN."

The host church placed Vicky and the family on the front row. Vicky's bottom was sore, and her back was hurting during the concert. But, Vicky was determined to visit with Karen. Half way through the concert Vicky got hot, and she took off her wig. At the beginning of the last song, Karen introduced Vicky Bowen (also known as Sassy) to the entire audience. Vicky responded to the warm welcome with tears of joy. After the concert, many people came by and greeted Vicky, including the missionary, Shannon Buckner. Karen's manager, Dick, escorted the family back to see Karen. Vicky asked if Shannon could go with her. Karen, Shannon, and Vicky visited for quite a while. After Shannon left, Karen and Vicky talked about the cancer treatments, Christmas, the upcoming prom, and graduation. Vicky was thrilled to visit with Karen again. Vicky was encouraged to keep up the battle against cancer. Vicky played Karen's CDs all the way back to the apartment.

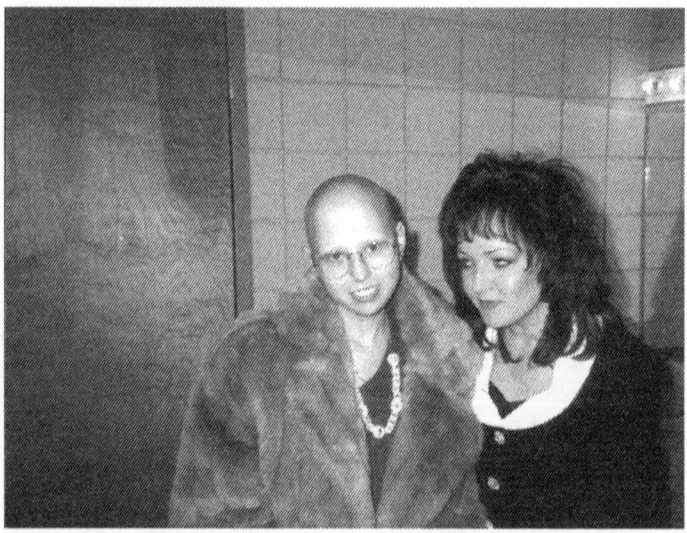

Vicky visiting with Karen Wheaton.

MORE RADIATION

Vicky ate a few bites of cheese and lunch meat before the family drove home Saturday. Vanessa and I needed to go home for additional medical supplies. Vicky stayed home with Vanessa Sunday morning because of severe nausea. With the help of her medication, Vicky was able to keep down half of a honey bun for breakfast. I packed the car after church, and Vicky laid back to sleep for the trip to Little Rock. Back at the apartment, Vicky was much more alert. She helped put away the medical supplies and her clothes. She ate cheese and lunchmeat for dinner before working on crafts. Vicky worked for hours on the crafts sent to her by those who wanted to encourage Vicky.

On Monday morning, Vanessa and I took Vicky to CARTI to evaluate radiation to the other bones cancer was located in. Vicky became nauseated while waiting and started bleeding from her nose. Vicky lay on her back to stop the bleeding. All of the bone scans for this year were clear. The bone scans obtained in June of the previous year showed one vertebra and the left hip socket having cancer. The MRI scans did not show any soft tumors growing out of these bones. Doctor Stine, at Arkansas Children's Hospital wanted to include the original scans taken in 1995 for treatment. From all of the scans, the treatment would consist of 25 exposures of radiation over 5 weeks. Doctor Harris, at CARTI, told Vicky to start taking her nausea medicine on a routine basis in the morning and evening to get over the effects of nausea. She should get use to the sedating effects in a few days. Doctor Harris wanted to review the original reports from 1995 before starting treatments.

Vicky went to day medicine Tuesday for two units of red blood. Her platelets had decreased to 13, and she received a unit of platelets also. I spoke to Doctor Becton about Vicky's pills passing trough her intestinal tract so quickly. The doctor asked Vanessa and I to stop the stool softening pills until stool formed. Vicky could not hold her bowels when she pushed her IV pole to the bathroom, and she had to change into a hospital gown. Vincristine chemotherapy was administered while Vicky was in for transfusions. Vicky had no white blood cells and had to take precautions to keep from getting an infection. Vicky had to wear the hospital gown to the apartment.

On the way back to the apartment Vicky stopped at a video store to rent a movie about Reba McEntire. Cancer Care Inc. called Vicky to help her cope with her cancer and treatments. Cancer Care is a counseling organization for kids and adults with cancer. They pair the patient up to a person who had similar forms of cancer and treatments. The organization asked for some history on Vicky's cancer and treatments.

Vicky ate half of a honey bun before going to CARTI for her consultation Wednesday. Doctor Harris had reviewed all of the records, and Vicky needed treatments in both upper leg bones (femurs) and one of the lumbar vertebrae. Vicky was marked on her back and both legs with a red marker. She was scheduled to receive 25 treatments. The back would get 180 Rads of radiation each day. Each leg would get 90 Rads to the front and then 90 Rads to the back each day. This was a total of 4,140 Rads to each location for a total of 12,420 Rads over 25 days. This large amount of energy was needed to kill the cancer. Her appointments were scheduled for 1:00 each afternoon.

Vicky called Kara Travis at Arkansas Children's Hospital to see if she wanted lunch from Taco Bell. Kara asked for a soft taco and a Mexican pizza. Vicky delivered the food to Kara's room and then visited for fifteen minutes. The two girls compared notes on their treatments and then talked about boys. Vicky was scheduled to have her red wig styled at the St. Vincent hospital New Outlook program Thursday. The two girls compared wigs before Vicky left for the apartment. Vicky became very emotional when she saw how much of her body was marked for radiation. She was crying most of the night and wanted Mom and I to hold her. Vicky went to bed with us without taking her evening pills.

Vicky was moving very slowly when she woke up Thursday morning. She ate a few bites for breakfast and threw it back up. When she stood to walk, she was very light headed. Vanessa and I took Vicky to have her wig styled after her radiation treatment. Vicky said she was too tired to go and did not care what her wig looked like. I made Vicky get up and go to the car. The wig was beautiful, and her face was made-up with red eyebrows that matched the wig, but all Vicky wanted to do was go back to the apartment to lay down. I traveled home on the CMS van to pick up my car while Vanessa took Vicky to the apartment. At first, Vicky wanted the feed tube inserted, but she agreed to try eating popsicles and Jell-O.

Terry left my car packed with feed tube equipment and the mail. I drove back to Little Rock during the night. Vicky received a picture from Reba McEntire, and she stayed up most of the night looking at the picture while listening to her music. Vicky wanted to meet Reba one day.

I went back to work on Friday the 24th, and home health came to the apartment to check Vicky's blood counts. Vicky's port site was tender, and she asked the nurse to draw blood from her arm. Vicky's veins were so small and deep that it was hard to draw blood. The blood test results showed her platelet count at 4. Doctor Becton called, and told Vanessa to take Vicky to the emergency room at Children's Hospital for a platelet transfusion as soon as the CARTI treatment was completed. The emergency room staff immediately sent Vicky over to day medicine because of the large number of sick kids in the emergency room. Vicky received one unit of platelets. A boy who survived Ewing's sarcoma called Vicky in the evening and spoke with her for 40 minutes. The survivor, Patrick, called Vicky back Monday night to talk again. Vicky felt much better having talked with others who where in the same situation.

Vicky started crying when she went to bed, stating that she missed all of her school friends.

Vicky's mouth sores were getting worse, and she did not want to eat dinner Friday night. She asked me to put in the feed tube. Vicky held onto her small bucket and box of tissue while I lubricated the new feed tube. Vicky asked to put the tube in herself. Vicky took a deep breath as she started the tube down the left side of her nose. As the tube moved to the back of her throat, Vicky's eyes stated to flow with tears. She swallowed quickly as she moved the tube deeper and deeper into her stomach. Vicky rolled to her side as she started to gag, and panted with short breaths. Her big blue eyes were full of tears when she asked me if the tube was deep enough. Vicky pushed the tube in four more inches, and I then taped the tube to her nose. Vicky smiled, and said that she was getting pretty good at taking care of herself. I connected the tube to the equipment and ran the liquid feeds at a rate of 150 milliliters per hour.

Saturday morning I put two containers of liquid feed through Vicky's feed tube at a rate of 300 milliliters per hour. Vicky then capped the feed tube and asked to go to McDonalds for lunch. Vicky was very weak, but she made the walk up the stairs to the car. When Vicky walked into McDonalds she instantly became nauseated from the smell of hamburgers cooking, and she had to go back to the car. Vanessa stayed with Vicky while I picked up Happy Meals for Stacy and Windle. Vicky would not let Windle and Stacy eat in the car because of the smell making her sick. Vicky did not eat any lunch. She asked to shop at K-Mart. Vicky became nauseated again and left after buying a card for her nurse, Rhonda. Vicky was very tired and asked to go back to the apartment.

When Vicky did her mouth care, there was fresh blood in her mouth. She started crying because of the pain from the mouth sores. She became nauseated and asked for medication to calm her stomach. I gave Vicky her medications through the feed tube, and she went to sleep. I connected the feed tube to the pump and started the liquid feeds at 150 milliliters per hour.

Vanessa's leg started hurting again Saturday. Vanessa called Sister Sheila, and talked for a while. Sister Sheila asked to talk with Vicky, but Vicky didn't feel like talking to anyone because her mouth hurt so badly. I checked Vicky's temperature, and it was normal. Vicky had to hurt badly when she did not want to talk with Sister Sheila.

I checked Vicky's temperature again Sunday morning, and it was still normal. I took Windle and Stacy to the Ferndale Assembly of God church just south of Little Rock. The church was very friendly and wanted to pray for Vicky and the family. When the kids and I returned from church Vicky was up watching television. I helped Vicky to clean her mouth. Her tongue was completely covered white with thrush.

Every time Vicky had a bowel movement, she had stomach cramps and became nauseated. I gave her medication for the nausea, and Vicky took a nap. I woke her up in the evening, and did the mouth care again. Stacy started having diarrhea, and Vanessa and I were concerned if there was any connections with Vicky's stomach cramping. I checked Vicky's temperature, and it was 100.9 degrees. Vicky started crying thinking that she was sick and would have to go into the hospital. I checked the temperature again one hour later, and it had dropped to 99.3 degrees. Vicky asked to sleep with Mom and I Sunday night. She wanted Mom to hold her hand while I rubbed her back. I started the liquid feeds at 150 milliliters per hour again. I had to grind up all of Vicky's pills in order to put them down the feed tube. Vicky was up every two hours to use the bathroom. Vicky's eyes welled with tears each time her stomach cramped. You could hear Vicky crying over the sound of the wind outside.

I checked Vicky's temperature Monday morning before going to work, and it was 99.5 degrees. The 90-minute ride to work was especially hard on me. Close to work the muffler fell off of the car. I called Terry, and had him pick the car up to have the muffler replaced. Home health came to the apartment to check Vicky's blood counts.

My coworkers sent money and gifts home to help lift Vicky's spirits. Vicky asked to go to Wal Mart where she placed a bathing suit on layaway. It was amazing how much more alert and better feeling Vicky was after receiving the gifts. I realized that lifting the spirits of a child with cancer had just as much effect as a blood transfusion. Vicky was hooked back up to the liquid feeds at bedtime. Vicky wanted to sleep in her own bed with her Taz pillow. She slept peacefully all night. Vicky woke up feeling much better in the morning. At CARTI Vicky decided she wanted to start eating. She slowly picked at the tape one her nose, and then pulled the feed tube out. My eyes watered just from watching Vicky pull the feed tube out. Vicky slowly swallowed all of her pills by mouth.

I ate lunch at work with Terry Tuesday. Terry brought the mail to me, and in it was a notice of foreclosure from the Veteran's Administration. I sent copies of Vicky's journals to the mortgage company and the Veteran's Administration. I then called Gregg Adams at Arkansas Children's hospital and asked if there was any financial assistance available. Gregg mailed an application for assistance to the apartment. Vicky worked on crafts, and Patrick called from New Jersey. Vicky and Patrick talked about chemotherapy and radiation treatments for over 30 minutes. Vanessa was used to me putting Vicky's pills down the feed tube before I left for work, but Vicky no longer had a tube into her stomach. I noticed the pills were still on the counter when I arrived at the apartment after work. Vicky took her morning pills for me, and then asked to go out to a Mexican restaurant for dinner. She ate a few bites of a cheese enchilada, a few bites of beans, and several chips with cheese dip. All of her dinner stayed down. Vicky then asked to go to Wal-Mart to buy a dress for church. Vicky asked if the family could go home for the weekend. She wanted to see Johnna Boone and Sister Sheila. Vicky asked to pay for the dress herself, but she was short $10.00. Vicky started laughing as she left the register stating that she beat me out of $10.00. It was great to see Vicky acting so "Sassy." Terry called the apartment just as Vanessa and I went to bed. Terry called to say that he had to buy some groceries, and was running out of food. He stated that one of the lights was out on his car. Vanessa got angry with me for falling asleep after talking with Terry. She wanted me stay awake to talk, but I was very tired. I was only getting five hours of sleep each night and driving an hour and a half to and from work. My arm started feeling numb again because of all of the stress.

The home health nurse came to the apartment Thursday morning for Vicky's blood test. The clinic called with the results and asked Vanessa to take Vicky to the hospital after radiation treatments to direct admit into the hospital for a red blood transfusion. Jack Glaze, and his family, were in Little Rock. They called to visit Vicky, but she had to be at CARTI and the hospital. Doctor Harris told Vicky at CARTI that she needed to drink a minimum of eight glasses of water each day to help with diarrhea. He gave Vicky pain medication to help with back pain caused by radiation to the vertebrae. I drove to the hospital after work so Vanessa could take Windle and Stacy to the apartment. Doctor Saylors, at Arkansas Children's hospital, stated that when bone marrow is killed by radiation, red blood fills in the space. This was why Vicky's red blood count dropped so quickly during radiation treatment to the bones. I went to the apartment after the "Hip Police" started the transfusion. Nurse "Hip Police" was pregnant, and was due the first of August. Vicky had transfused a total of 97 units of red blood, 75 units of platelets, and 7 units of plasma since being diagnosed with cancer. Her first transfusion was January 16 of last year.

I put Windle on the school bus Friday morning at the apartment, and then went to the hospital. Vicky was doing very well. She ate Jell-O with fruit for breakfast. Vicky checked out of the hospital at 10:00 a.m. and went to CARTI. Vicky asked to eat lunch at Backyard Barbecue. She ate french fries and ice cream. The family left Little Rock and went home when Windle returned from school. On the drive home Vicky ate some lunchmeat and cheese. Vicky asked to eat dinner at a restaurant where two of her friends worked. Vicky ate a bite of hamburger, a bite from a cheese sandwich, several onion rings, and a few tatter tots. Vicky talked to her friends about school, graduation, and the Prom. Vicky called and talked with Sister Sheila before going to bed. Vicky called for me because her back was hurting. Vicky was crying because of the pain. She asked to have her back and left shoulder rubbed. Vicky curled up with the bunny that her nurse, Rhonda Best, got her for Easter. Vicky cried herself to sleep.

Terry asked me to go to the shooting range with him Saturday morning. I knew that I needed to spend time with Terry also. Vicky asked to eat lunch with Terry. Vicky, Terry, and I went to Lazy Earl's truck stop for lunch. Vicky ate mashed potatoes with white gravy; onion rings, french fries, and sliced dill pickles. Vanessa and I took Terry to the grocery store, and bought food for a month. The whole family went to visit with Brother Dade and Sister Sheila. On the way home Vicky picked up the ingredients for a Mexican dinner. Vanessa, Windle, and Stacy went to Wal Mart while Vicky and I made dinner. Vicky ate a burrito, and then snacked on cream cheese. Vicky's shoulder hurt more than her back when she went to bed.

Sunday, February 2, was my birthday. Vicky asked me if I would help her to play a tape at church. At church, Vicky gave a testimony how prayers and support changed her health this week. I then played the Ricky Skaggs song; "Somebody's Praying." Everyone in church was excited to see Vicky doing so well. For lunch, Vicky took me to Lazy Earl's truck stop for my birthday. Vicky ate the same foods she did the day before. The family packed up, and went back to the apartment in Little Rock. My sister, Barbara, called for my birthday. She also talked with Vicky. Vicky called Sister Sheila, and then she called Kara Travis. Kara was going into the hospital Monday for chemotherapy. Vicky then worked on her homework.

A home health nurse came to the apartment Monday morning for Vicky's blood work. The results were very good. Gregg Adams called me with financial assistance through Children's Cancer Society. I passed the information on to the mortgage company. Vicky went to the hospital to visit with Kara for her birthday. Vicky bought matching purses for her and Kara, and made friendship bracelets. Kara was on special IV fluids for nutrition, and went from 90 to 108 pounds. Vicky and Kara had a good time. Vicky was very upbeat all day. She ate a burrito with cheese just before going to bed at midnight.

Carol Godfrey called from Clinic 3 Tuesday morning. Doctor Stine wanted Vicky to start chemotherapy on Friday following her radiation treatment. Vicky contacted CARTI and registered to meet with the PALS the following Monday at Luby's cafeteria. PALS is a group of people who spend time with cancer patients. Vicky asked to have onion rings for dinner.

CARTI asked Vicky to come up with a list of gifts. Vicky would receive one or more of these items when she finished her radiation treatments. CARTI changed Vicky's Friday appointment to 7:30 a.m. so that she could be at Clinic 3 by 9:00 a.m. to start chemotherapy. Terry delivered the mail to me at work. In the mail were the renewal forms for Vicky's Medicaid. Vicky was feeling very sad and called Sister Sheila to talk for a while. The two talked for a long time. Vicky then asked me to make an appointment with the hospital chaplain and Gregg Adams on Friday. Vicky wanted to talk about her feelings about cancer because she was tired of hurting so much. Vicky asked for a pain pill and asked me to rub her left shoulder blade and tailbone. Vicky finally cried herself to sleep.

I called Clinic 3 Thursday morning to get the results of the morning blood tests. Vicky might have to delay chemotherapy because of so many new cancer patients during the week. I told the nurse that Vicky wanted to speak with the chaplain and Gregg Adams about her feelings. At CARTI, Vicky picked out a doll from their gift closet. She then turned in her list of gifts she wanted. There was a package at the apartment for Vicky from her Aunt Jackie. In the package was a book by Billy Graham about angels. Vicky read the book all evening. I asked if I could read the book when Vicky was finished.

Vicky went to CARTI early Friday morning and then on to Clinic 3. Cynthia was one of the clinic nurses. She said that she was at the Karen Wheaton concert in Conway the same time Vicky was there. Cynthia asked if Vicky would let her know when Karen would be in concert again. Cynthia asked Vicky if she wanted her port accessed. Vicky asked to have her blood test in the arm, and then access her port in the hospital later. Vicky was admitted to room 3123 for chemotherapy. I provided a list of medications to the clinic. The list now filled a full page. Vicky sent me to the store for her meals. She wanted frozen chicken burritos, sliced sweet pickles, and creme cheese.

I stopped by the blood bank to ask a question about blood types. I found out that red blood cells could have up to three antigens attached to them. These are called antigens A, B, and D. If the blood cell has antigen A attached to it, it is type A blood. If antigen B is attached, it is type B blood. When both antigens A and B are attached, it is type AB blood. The absence of both antigens A and B is type O blood. When antigen D is present, the blood is Rh-positive. The absence of antigen D is Rh-negative. If a person is Rh negative (no D antigen), they cannot have Rh-positive blood. Type O, Rh-negative blood is considered universal. If the patient is transfused with blood that has an antigen that the patient does not have, there could be a severe reaction.

The hospital chaplain, John, came to visit with Vicky Friday afternoon. The two spoke in private for an hour. Chemotherapy was started in the evening. Vicky called the apartment and asked for her sheep skin throw to lay on.

Vanessa and I met another family Saturday who had a daughter with cancer. Their daughter finished her second round of chemotherapy and had spiked a fever. I shared Vicky's notebook with the family. Vicky checked on Kara, and she was having trouble with her stomach. Vicky asked me to give a picture to Kara to cheer her up. It was a picture of the two together when they visited in the hospital last time. I mentioned that Wal Mart could copy the picture onto T-shirts. Vicky liked the idea, and wrote out a slogan to put with the picture. "CANCER—been there. CHEMO—done that. Got the VICTORY!" The nurses were going to sign the T-shirts, and then present them to both Vicky and Kara.

Vicky received three forms of chemotherapy this time. There was one round of cytoxin, one round of vinchristine, and three rounds of VP-16. Vicky stated that she was feeling "chemo puny." She said that it means that she would like to give up, but knows to keep fighting. Vicky asked Mom to stay with her Saturday night.

I took Windle and Stacy to church Sunday morning, and then checked Vicky out of the hospital. Vicky asked if she could go watch a movie. I asked the theater manager if Vicky could go in first to limit the number of people she would be around. Vicky promised to wear her mask. Vicky ate lots of popcorn and candy during the show. Vicky wanted Mexican food for dinner, and she ate well. Vicky then asked to go to Wal Mart. She used the money given to her to buy a pretty white night gown. Vicky gave her own injection, and then checked on Kara. Kara was still in the hospital with severe nausea.

Home health came to the apartment Monday morning for blood work. I used Vicky's blood test history, and found that she would need transfusions by the weekend. The clinic scheduled Vicky for red blood and platelet transfusions on Friday. A woman at my work sent Vicky a pretty red heart bracelet. The woman had it blessed by her priest. Another person at my work sent a Mickey nightshirt. The family went to Terry Elementary for Windle's school program. Vicky finished typing her eleventh journal. She was very active and alert all day.

Jack Glaze called me Tuesday, and stated that his church had an offering for the family. One of my coworkers gave me a check for $25.00 to take to Vicky. Vicky spent the evening mailing her journals. There were one hundred addresses on her mailing list.

I rode to work Wednesday with a woman who lived in Little Rock. On the way home from work my arm and chest started to hurt. Vicky cashed her check Wednesday night and went to Wal Mart. She bought a Mickey Mouse tie to give to doctor Stine Friday. Vicky received a card from Sister Sheila and a stack of cards from her school. Vicky was feeling so well that she asked to eat at a Mexican restaurant again, but at dinner she became nauseated. Vanessa took Vicky to the bathroom to clean up. On the way home, Vicky became light headed and dizzy. Vicky called Gregg Adams at home, and talked with him for a long time. She then called Sister Sheila. Vicky asked to go into the hospital a day early for transfusions. She said that she could tell that her red blood count was real low.

It snowed six inches in Little Rock early Thursday morning. I did not go to work, and home health was snow bound. I took Vicky to Children's Hospital for her blood work and then to CARTI for her radiation treatment. Clinic 3 called CARTI, and told Vicky to return to the hospital for a direct admission because her blood counts were low. Vanessa delivered a blanket she made for Vicky's nurse, Janet. Vicky gave the Mickey Mouse tie to Carol Godfrey to deliver to doctor Stine. The nurse at the desk noticed that Vicky's arm was bleeding. The gauze over the site of the blood test was soaked in blood. It was obvious that Vicky needed platelets. Vicky was admitted to room 3131 for three units of red blood, two units of platelets, and her vinchristine chemotherapy. Kara was still in the hospital, and she was very lonely. The lining on Kara's throat was gone because of the constant nausea. She was on a morphine pump for the pain. I visited with Kara for over an hour. She wanted so much for someone to stay the night in the room with her. I would have stayed with Kara, but there were too many legal issues about her parent's consent. Vanessa stayed at the apartment with Windle and Stacy, and I stayed the night with Vicky.

I went to work from the hospital Friday morning. I checked Vicky out of the hospital after work. Her noon pills were still on the tray, and

I made Vicky take them. Vicky stopped to visit with Kara before leaving. Vicky stayed in the car while Vanessa and I packed, and then the family went home for the weekend. There was a message from Kara on the answering machine when Vicky got home. Vicky called her back, and spoke for half an hour. Vicky needed pain medication for her back in order to go to sleep. I rubbed Vicky's back as feel asleep.

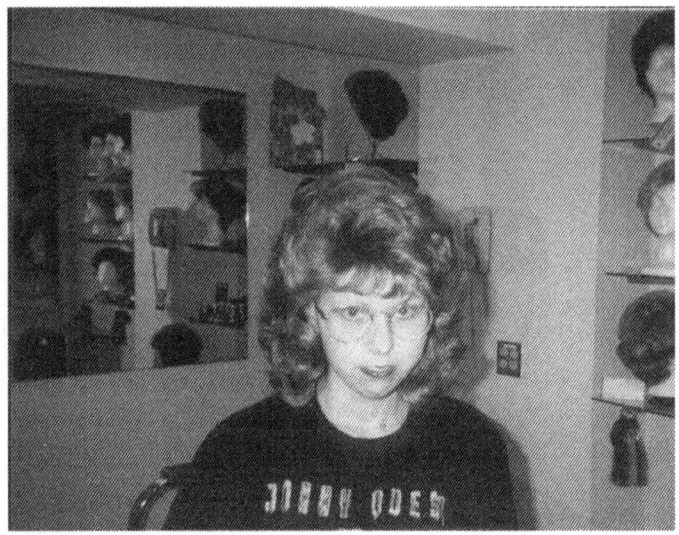

Vicky was not feeling well when this wig was styled.

Two Kids of Angels

I heard Vicky calling for me early Saturday morning. Vicky was hungry at 2:30 in the morning, and wanted sweet pickles and cream cheese. She complained about her port site looking infected and hurting. I cleaned the area with Betadine and alcohol, and covered it with antibacterial cream. Vicky tried to swallow a sweet pickle, but there was too much pain. Her mouth was covered white with thrush, and one area was bleeding. I helped Vicky wash her mouth with her foam toothbrush in an attempt to remove the thrush. She stated that her throat and ears were sore. I checked her temperature, and it was 100.5 degrees.

Vicky said that she wanted Tylenol, but that she could not swallow her pills. She asked me to insert the feed tube in order to taker her medications, and let her throat rest. Vicky had trouble swallowing as the feed tube was inserted. Her eyes flooded with tears, she became nauseated, and the end of the tube came out of her mouth with the other end out of her nose. Vicky's eyes had a panic look as she did all she could to keep from gagging, but a large volume of liquids came up. I pulled the tube out slowly and tried again. It took two more attempts to get the feed tube all the way in. I ground up Vicky's Tylenol, and medication for her nausea. She went back to bed, and slept for several hours. I cleaned up the mess on Vicky's floor.

Vicky's temperature was checked when she woke up, and it was 101.3 degrees. I called Children's Hospital, and spoke with doctor Stine. Vicky needed to go to the emergency room right away. Vanessa and I packed the car, and headed for Little Rock.

Vicky was started on Fortaz antibiotic and given medication for nausea. Liquid feeds were started at 120 milliliters for 12 hours each night. The blood test showed that Vicky needed one unit of platelets. One liter of fluids and the platelets were administered in the emergency room. Vicky started to complain about the hard beds hurting her back. Vicky was placed in room 3127 just after midnight where she slept well all night. I took Windle and Stacy to the apartment while Vanessa stayed with Vicky.

I called the pastor, brother Dade, before service Sunday morning, and asked for prayer cloths for both Vicky and Kara. Vicky woke up in the morning with nausea. Her feed tube plugged up, and it could not be cleared. Vicky asked for the feed tube to be replaced because she could not swallow any pills. Her throat was still very raw and extremely sore. The nurse put the new feed tube down the other side of Vicky's nose in order to reduce the irritation. Doctor Stine checked in on Vicky, and thanked her for the special tie. Vicky's blood test showed her white blood count to be zero.

The blood test Monday morning showed Vicky's white blood count still at zero. The carbon dioxide level in the blood was moving in the acid direction. My records showed the carbon dioxide level dropping from 27 to 19 over the past two months. The alkaphos and phosphorus levels were also very low. Alkaphos is the measure of an enzyme output from the gut and bones. Phosphorus is an element required for normal cell function. Vicky was taken off of Jevity liquid feeds through the feed tube, and placed on special IV food through her IV port. This allowed Vicky's throat and stomach to rest. The feed tube was used for medications only. The blood cultures were still negative for any infection of the blood system. Vicky started having a deep cough, and the doctors considered requesting a chest x-ray.

I put Windle on the bus for school Tuesday morning, and then placed Stacy in day care before going to work. Debbie Cole and Georgia watched Stacy for a few days. Vicky's blood test was performed twice during the day to verify equilibrium using the IV line for nutrition. Vicky maintained a mild cough all day along with nausea. Vicky's bed had to be changed several times.

Vicky asked to have something to eat, but she was told "no" because of the open ulcers and thrush in her mouth. Vicky convinced herself that she was headed for PICU. Vicky started crying as thoughts of dying filled her mind. She became combative with Vanessa and the nurses in an attempt to be "Sassy." More than anything Vicky wanted to live. The only way she knew to do so was to keep "Sassy" alive. Gregg Adams stopped by to speak with Vicky. She told Gregg that she knew she would die if she went to intensive care. She was worried because she could no longer tolerate liquid feeds on her stomach, and that nutrition through the IV had to be started. She was also worried because her temperature was still going up. Gregg convinced Vicky that there is a big difference between keeping "Sassy" alive and being abusive. Vicky apologized to Mom and the nurses. A young youth minister by the name of Jason called to check on Vicky. He heard that Vicky was having a hard time dealing with her feelings. This youth minister also had cancer, and was taking chemotherapy. Jason asked if he and his mom could visit with Vicky on Wednesday. Vicky needed another unit of red blood transfused in the evening.

Vicky needed another unit of red blood early Wednesday morning. When the nursed checked on Vicky, her weight was 103.6 pounds, and her temperature was 103.2 degrees. Vicky became nauseated has she tried to get back in bed. The nurses sat her in the rocking chair, and changed the bedding. Vicky was given Tylenol and a bed bath to lower the temperature. All of the morning medications were put down the feed tube, and stayed down. A x-ray of the lungs showed that the lower left lobe was diminished.

Fluconizole, an antifungal was started for the thrush in Vicky's mouth. Vicky's temperature spiked to 104.4 degrees, and her mouth was hurting badly again. Vicky started begging the nurses for morphine to control the pain. The youth pastor, Jason, and his mom visited with Vicky. She also received a bouquet of flowers from the TLC foundation. I relieved Vanessa for the night. Vicky asked me to do therapy on the lower left lung. I placed a towel over Vicky's back, and started patting the towel. Vicky then took deep breaths and coughed. Vicky asked for this treatment several times during the night. I was willing to stay up all night with Vicky to help keep "Sassy" alive. Vicky asked me to mail a letter with pictures to Karen Wheaton.

I ate breakfast Thursday morning with Kara and her mom. One of Kara's feet was swelling with a skin infection. Vanessa came to the hospital after Windle went to school. Vicky's blood counts showed her white count was still at zero. The carbon dioxide level had dropped to 13, and all of the other blood counts looked real good. The dietitian wanted to start feeds into the stomach during the night at 50 milliliters per hour. The pain team was called in, and Vicky was allowed to have morphine every two to four hours as needed. Vicky needed two units of red blood. After the first unit was transfused, Vicky ran a fever, and the second unit was put on hold. Again Vicky was overwhelmed with the fear of dying because of the fever. Vicky became angry and argued with her nurse. When Vanessa tried to scold Vicky, she hit Mom.

When Vicky's fever came down, the second unit of red blood was transfused early Friday morning. Vicky's port clotted while the nurses were trying to get the morning blood samples. Carol Godfrey put in a special medication to remove the clot, and Vicky's right arm was accessed for her IV lines. The area over Vicky's implanted port started bleeding. Her mouth ulcers also started bleeding. Vicky's blood pressure dropped, and she became very disoriented, and then unresponsive. "Sassy" was dying. The doctor ordered one-on-one nursing care, and two units of platelets were pushed. The quick action of the nurses who remembered this same scenario a year ago saved Vicky from a trip to intensive care. The pediatrician was very responsive to the input from the nurses, Vanessa and I, and Vicky. The thrush (yeast infection) was advancing down Vicky's throat to her lungs when it was put in check with the antifungal called Fluconizole.

Vicky's blood pressure slowly recovered, and she became alert again. She complained that her rectum was hurting. The nurse checked, and the area was swollen, and very red. The doctor ordered a urinalysis and another lung x-ray. Vicky's white blood count was still at zero. Vicky's central line cleared of the blood clot, and the lines were removed from Vicky's arm.

Gregg Adams was called in to talk with Vicky about how she was dealing with her fear of dying. Gregg asked to talk with Vicky, Vanessa, and I again later on. Vicky needed to understand that it was OK to be angry, but that there are right and wrong ways to vent that anger. Kara's mom told Vanessa and I that Kara had surgery today to install a new central line that would allow for harvesting of Kara's stem cells for a possible bone marrow transplant.

After Vicky was stable, I went to Victoria's Secret, and picked up a nightgown and underwear Vicky identified in a catalog. The nurse assistant, Barbara, helped Vicky with a bath. She then put the new nightgown on Vicky. Vicky claimed that she was the "Babe of Hawaii" in her new nightgown. When Vanessa went back to the apartment, Vicky called her. Vicky wanted to let Mom know that she was feeling much better, and not to worry. Vicky then asked me to record the following information about angels that she saw when her blood pressure dropped.

"When my blood pressure dropped, Windle was sent out of the room, and Mom went out with him. On the left side of my room (by the closet door) angels of Satan were piling up. The same amount of angels came on the right side, but they were God's angels. There was the sound of a whistle. Each side tried to amass angels. As a bell sounded, the right side of my room was filled with an innumerable amount of God's angels compared to only 10 of Satan's angels. Then a voice from inside my ear (and coming from the right side of the room) said, "Have no fear for everything is in control." For some unknown reason, someone was tugging at

me to rebuke the demons. When I did, they all went away. The number of God's angels doubled on the whole wall. The angels of God then went away. Every now and then two or three of God's angels came into the room, walked back and forth, and then were gone. This occurred about every fifteen minutes.

Then there was the light sound of angels playing Amazing Grace. The sound became louder and louder. The angels all came from the wall one by one around my bed. The one head angel reached out to me and spoke some kind of prayer. I remember passing out. The next thing I remember was Dad walking into the room at 9:00 p.m. The angels were friendly and fun to be around. They reassured me that if I needed them, they would be right there for me."

Vicky was placed on a morphine pump Saturday morning. The pump delivered a set background dose, and additional morphine was delivered when Vicky pushed a button. Vicky pushed the button every hour. The morning blood count showed that Vicky's white blood count was starting to increase. Brother Dade came to visit with Vicky. Vicky told him about her visit with the angels the day before. Vanessa and I visited with another family, whose fifteen-year-old son had Ewing's Sarcoma, while Brother Dade and Vicky talked about her anger.

Vicky's feed tube plugged Sunday morning. Vicky asked if she could remove the old feed tube and insert the new one herself. Vicky's nurse watched as Vicky completed the task on her own. While Vicky was washing her tongue, the ulcers started bleeding. The doctor told Vicky that she had to stop scrubbing her tongue, and do the "swish and spit" routine. The morning blood test showed that Vicky's white count had doubled from the day before, but she could still get an infection. Another unit of platelets was transfused to control the bleeding. I took Windle and Stacy to Church in the morning, and Vanessa took Windle and Stacy to the apartment in the evening. Vicky wanted her own night-gown instead of a hospital gown after her bath. Vicky always felt better about herself when she dressed up.

Vicky transfused another unit of platelets Monday morning because of fresh blood in her mouth. Vicky received the largest get-well poster anyone had ever seen from the Bentonville Assembly of God youth group. Vicky was feeling so much better that her morphine pump background setting was cut in half and Vicky told her nurse that she wanted to give her own injection. Liquid feeds were increased up to 150 milliliters per hour during the night. Vicky' weight was up to 107.5 pounds. Kara called and checked on Vicky. Kara started the procedure for stem cell harvesting.

Vicky didn't sleep well during the night. She woke up after only four hours of rest with a temperature of 104 degrees. Her mouth was really sore again, and she had to push the button on the morphine pump several times. Vicky tolerated the feeds at 150 milliliters during the night. Vicky's temperature returned to normal and then went back up to 102.6 degrees. More Tylenol was needed. Vicky transfused two more units of red blood. Brother Dade came and visited with Vicky and Kara.

A blood drive was held at my work on the 26th, and it was dedicated to Vicky. The mailbox at the apartment was stuffed with cards and letters to Vicky. She was so excited to read all of the wonderful words of encouragement from everyone. Vicky was feeling much better, and her morphine pump background setting was cut in half again. CARTI sent Vicky an invitation to go to Las Vegas, and she was getting excited about flying to Nevada.

The background setting on the morphine pump was set to zero Thursday morning. Vicky's right eye was red and swollen with an infection. She was given an antibiotic to put into her eye, and Vicky was willing to do anything to stop the itch. Vicky received a lot of mail from several Assembly of God youth groups, and from all of the kids at Stacy's day care. Vicky was feeling so well that she asked Vanessa and I to go to the apartment so she could spend time alone with her nurses.

Vicky was released from the hospital Friday morning after a platelet transfusion. I made arrangements to have a feed pump delivered to the apartment. CARTI was scheduled to reevaluate radiation treatments Monday afternoon. Carol Godfrey set Vicky up with an appointment Wednesday at Clinic 3 for the last round of chemotherapy. Vicky's blood counts would be checked by home health Monday to see if chemotherapy had to be delayed. When Vicky arrived at the apartment, she asked to check the mail. She had a handbag from her aunt Barbara, a musical angel from aunt Jackie, and a special letter from Karen Wheaton. Vicky asked to go shopping at the mall. She found a beautiful dress for Easter. Vicky still had a cough and I made her wear her mask.

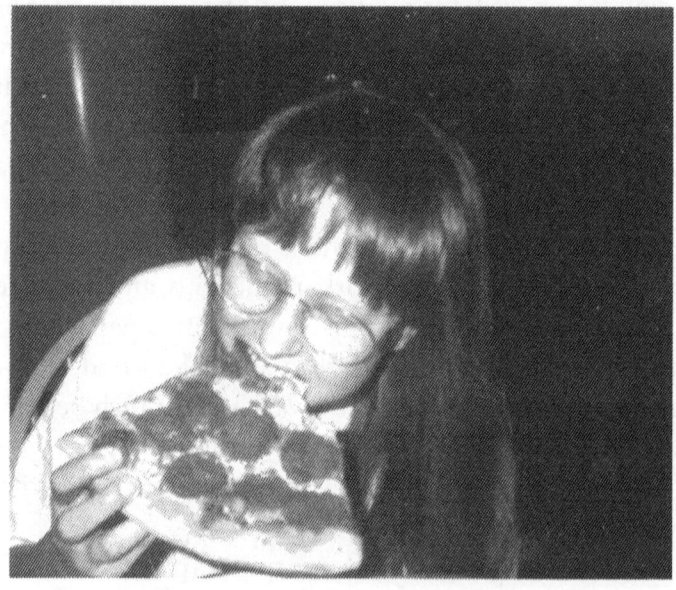

Vicky is eating her favorite meal of pizza.

A LUNG BIOPSY

The first weekend in March found Vicky shopping for cloths at Wal Mart. She was required to wear her mask at all times to keep from catching any illness. Vicky was still coughing after her recent trip to the hospital.

A home health nurse came to the apartment for Vicky's blood test Monday morning. The nurse noted that Vicky still had a rough cough. Vanessa took Vicky to CARTI in the afternoon to evaluate restarting the radiation treatments. The platelet level was 18, and the doctor would not start radiation with it this low. The white count was also low as if Vicky was fighting off an infection. Vicky was back at the apartment when Windle returned from school.

Vicky woke up early Tuesday morning feeling cold, and complaining that she could not get warm. I checked her temperature, and it was 99.8 degrees. I called the oncology doctor, and Vicky was scheduled for one unit of platelets in day medicine. X-rays of Vicky's lungs and sinus was taken while at the hospital. Carol Godfrey was not aware that CARTI was holding radiation for platelet levels. Doctor Stine called CARTI and scheduled Vicky to restart radiation on Thursday. Carol stated that the last round of chemotherapy would be administered when Vicky's platelet level was 40 to 50. Doctor Saylors checked Vicky and placed her on an antibiotic. He stated that her lungs are the best they had looked in a long time. Vicky did have sinus drainage on one side.

Vicky checked the mail when she got back to the apartment. There was a beautiful bathroom basket from a church youth group. Vicky received another package Wednesday from a Fort Smith youth group.

She was grateful knowing that other kids her age cared about her well being. Vicky wanted to know if she could go to all of these churches to express her appreciation to the youth.

Vanessa and Vicky returned to CARTI Thursday afternoon. Vicky was put back on the simulators and marked again. Vicky did not like all of the red markings on her legs and back, but she knew they were necessary. I had an appointment with a psychologist, and started taking Zoloft to help with my stress.

I worked until noon Friday and then took Vicky to CARTI for her radiation treatment. Vicky was in an argumentative mood and could not get along with anyone. Vanessa met Windle when he got home from school and packed for the weekend trip home. On the way home, Vicky said that she was getting nauseated. She asked me to stop the car and get her bucket. After a moment Vicky said the sensation was not nausea, but hunger. She laughed and started picking at the tape on her nose, and then pulled out the feed tube. Vicky started making plans for dinner and said she wanted Terry to join us for dinner at Lazy Earl's truck stop.

Vicky asked to try a chili cheese hot dog Saturday. She liked it so much that she wanted another one Sunday after church. When the family arrived back at the apartment Sunday evening there was a message on the answering machine from Kara Travis. Vicky called Kara, and the two talked for a long time. A boy Kara knew died of leukemia Thursday. As Vicky got up from the chair, she tripped on the phone cord. Her left knee bruised, her arms had red spots, her lip was bleeding, and her left earring hole was bleeding. Vicky lay on the couch crying as Vanessa helped stop the bleeding. I placed cold packs on the bruised areas. It was obvious that Vicky's platelet level was low. Vicky's cough was getting worse, especially while crying. Vicky did not want to go to the hospital to have her leg checked.

On Monday, March 10, the home health nurse found Vicky's temperature at 103.3, and blood pressure was low. Vanessa and I immediately took Vicky to Clinic 3. Vicky was admitted to the hospital for low blood counts, and possible pneumonia. Antibiotics for a bacterial pneumonia were started, and x-rays of the chest and left knee were obtained. One unit of platelets was transfused.

On Tuesday, Hillary Clinton came to Arkansas Children's hospital for the dedication of the new eye clinic. Kara and Vicky were invited to the ceremony, and they were able to meet the President's wife. The two teens used the time to catch up on their personal lives. Both girls were in their wheel chairs with their blue buckets. Vicky then went for a CT scan while Kara returned to her room. The visit by the First Lady was covered by the TV stations and was on the nightly news.

I was at work Tuesday teaching a class when Gregg Adams called. He said that it was an emergency. Doctor Stine performed a CT scan on Vicky after reviewing the chest x-ray. The results showed lumps in both of Vicky's lungs. There were lumps outside the lungs, between the lung and lung lining, and inside the lungs. I pressed Gregg for a verdict. Gregg stated that the prognosis was very poor. I had to be at the hospital before 6:00 for a consultation.

My coworkers picked up my workload, and I asked for a week off from work. I shared the report with my manager, and she asked me to wait a moment. She gave me a stuffed frog she was given recently to cheer herself up. She stated that I needed it more than she did. I put the frog on the dash of the car and then picked up Stacy from day care. There was so much to think about as I drove to Little Rock, but Stacy wanted to talk about school and the frog. I allowed Stacy to have priority.

Stacy and Windle went to the hospital playroom while Vanessa and I spoke with Doctor Stine and Gregg Adams. Surgery was scheduled for noon Wednesday to biopsy the left lung. Vicky would receive lots of platelets prior to the surgery to control bleeding. The surgeon would spread apart two ribs to get to the left lung. A special ventilator tube would go into each lung. The left lung would be collapsed, and the tumors would be sampled along with a piece of the lung. A chest tube would go into the top of the chest cavity to help the left lung inflate after surgery. The tube could come out after 24 hours if there was no bleeding. Once the tube was out Vicky would be required to start walking.

The doctor explained everything to Vicky after talking with Vanessa and I. Vicky was given a short life expectancy. Vicky requested to speak with her favorite nurse, Rhonda (the one Vicky nicknamed trashy). It was a quiet and depressing meeting, but Rhonda encouraged Vicky to have faith. Rhonda said that she would help Vicky fight to the end. Vicky called Sister Sheila and talked about the results of the tests. Brother Dade and Sister Sheila would be at the hospital for the surgery. Two units of platelets were transfused during the night.

Rhonda brought Vicky an angel vase Wednesday morning, and helped her to maintain a positive "Sassy" attitude. When Brother Dade and Sister Sheila arrived, they talked and prayed with Vicky.

The surgeon stopped by to explain the procedure to everyone. The lung is like a sponge wrapped in a lining that looks like saran wrap. When the biopsy of the lung is finished, a small titanium clip goes over the lung lining to seal off the incision. The chest tube is used to detect leaks from the incision. Antibiotics would be administered as a precaution. One unit of red blood would transfuse during the surgery.

As Vicky was rolled out of her room in route to surgery, I felt my legs give way to the weight of every emotion. I told Vanessa to go with Vicky, and I asked Gregg Adams to remain in the room. I slumped into the rocking chair as I felt every ounce of fight in me give way to pain and fear. Fifteen months of bottled up emotions were unleashed. Every physical feeling went numb as I cried at the impending loss of Vicky. Clutched in my hands was the stuffed frog.

For a short moment I was aware of Gregg's presence, but then the flood of tears came forth uncontrollably. In a short moment of control, I realized that the chaplain, John, was in the room. But, the wave of pain swallowed me up again. I was shaking uncontrollably, and my arms and legs went numb.

Then out of nowhere I was overwhelmed by a fear of death—my death. My ears echoed a muffled tone of my heart. The objects in the room blurred into a single foggy landscape. My arms and legs went limp. My heart ached like a strained muscle. Part of me wanted to give in, and escape any further hurt. I could see Gregg and John talking, but their words were worlds away.

Just then Brother Dade and Sister Sheila came to the doorway. I begged them to come in and help him. They prayed for me, but I was still numb to the natural surroundings. Then Brother Dade gave me a hug. I held on tight, and I could sense myself being pulled back to this world. The remainder of the day was like a dream for me that I could not escape. I realized that all of the day's events were out of my control. I felt so hopeless and useless. The only prayer I could summon was the one Windle and Stacy learned in Children's Church: "J, E, S, U, S, Jesus is the very best."

The surgeon came by to explain what he did. He removed tissue from three areas: the tumor mass; the lung, and material attached to the rib. A frozen section was not performed. The pathologist would check for bacteria, virus, and cancer cells. Doctor Stine stopped by also. He stated that the masses did not look good, and he expects cancer cells to be identified by the pathology department.

When Vicky returned to her room she was in a lot of pain. On a scale of 1 to 10, the pain was above a 10. When she coughed the pain went above 20, and tears welled up in both eyes. The nurses asked to have the morphine pump background setting increased. I spoke with Vicky about all of the options. Vicky said that she had already spoke with Rhonda about everything and she saw no choice but to fight. I stayed the night with Vicky, and Vanessa took Windle and Stacy to the apartment.

I was in a daze all day Thursday. Vanessa came to the hospital after Windle was put on the school bus. Brother Dade came to the hospital to attend a "Cancer Answers" program put on by CARTI. Brother Dade asked me to go with him. The class was held at a beautiful restaurant on the river. During the class several families agreed to pray for Vicky. I knew that it was raining, but I remembered very little about the presentation. The cloudy day was perfect for the way I was feeling. I knew that I needed to get away from the hospital with the pastor. I called my psychologist, and asked how to handle the stress. While I was trying to handle my stress, Vicky was having a very positive and enjoyable day.

I woke early Friday morning. As I was lying in Vicky's room the Lord gave me a vision which calmed my fears.

"I felt like I was on a small ship at sea in the midst of a storm. The ship had lost its rudder, and all means of propulsion. It was foggy and I knew land was not far away, but there were dangerous rocks to avoid. I was looking for the safety of a lighthouse where my journey started from, but there was no hint of any light. There were so many sounds around me, but none of them pointed to anything familiar. Then it dawned on me—there was a light coming from my vessel. There was a familiar small still voice next to me. The vessel I was on was sitting calm in the midst of the sea of storms. The water was softly knocking on the hull of the ship beneath the sounds of the storm. The Lord had always been on board with me. He is my captain and my friend. The fears subsided, and a sense of business filled my thoughts. It was time to get back to the business of preparing my vessel to set sail again. Then I remembered—we were leaving the harbor and heading into uncharted waters. We could not go back. Once this fog lifts (and it will) we will start moving again. My captain will make it clear to me one day where we are going and why. Until then I will remind myself that he is onboard, and in full control. There was nothing to fear but fear itself."

I took Windle and Stacy down to the cafeteria to eat breakfast. One of the cooks, Kent, gave Vicky a beautiful ceramic clown figurine. Sister Sheila came to visit Vicky and took her shopping in the hospital gift shop. Rhonda was Vicky's nurse again. Rhonda told Vicky that she would be gone for the next 10 days on a ski trip with her boyfriend. Vicky was having a great time joking with Rhonda about boyfriends.

Vicky told Rhonda not to expect an engagement ring, because the only ring she will every get is one around a bathtub. Vicky then opened a package from Sister Sheila that contained a Mickey Mouse T-shirt, Taz socks, and Mickey Mouse socks. Vicky's chest tube was removed with no signs of bleeding from the biopsy site.

I slept 10 hours, which helped me get fully rested. Doctor Stine came by the room Saturday morning with the biopsy results. He said that no tumor cells were found in any of the samples. Pieces of the lung lining that showed signs of thickening were removed during the biopsy. All of the samples looked like an infection, which was possibly a fungus. He stated that the results would be redone for verification. The infections control department wanted to do some special blood tests. A blood test for antibodies would be sent to the Mayo clinic for analysis. Doctor Stine had no idea where this infection came from. Treatment would consist of ampitericyn B as long as the masses respond as if it was a fungus. One unit of platelets was transfused to ensure that the wounds would not start bleeding. Vanessa took Windle and Stacy to Wal Mart and then to the apartment. I stayed the night with Vicky again. Vicky said that God had healer her of cancer in her lungs. During the night Vicky asked me to go to McDonald's for some chicken nuggets. She ate two of the nuggets before going to sleep at 3 in the morning.

Vicky's morphine pump was disconnected Sunday morning, and oral pain medication was started. Doctor Stine said that Friday's chest x-ray showed the masses responding to treatment. Vanessa, Vicky, Windle, Stacy, and I all went to Sunday school at the third floor play room.

Vicky's blood counts dropped more than expected Monday morning. She required two units of red blood and a unit of platelets. On Tuesday morning the blood counts were slightly better. Feeding through the IV was started because Vicky was not eating. Vicky visited the teen playroom in the evening. She spent an hour working on sand art. She was very good at the meticulous work, but she tired before she could finish. Vicky took the artwork back to her room to work on during the night.

Vicky's grandparents called from Texas. They were traveling from California and planned to visit on Easter weekend.

Vicky attended the spring gala Tuesday. She made an Easter basket. Vicky took so much time on the basket that the child life staff made her hat. Vicky was not happy. She wanted the gala to stay open longer. She wanted to make her own hat, but she was too tired. Vicky had a bite of ice cream before going back to her room.

Back at the room it was time for Vicky to take her pills. The nurse would not let Vicky stall. Lekretia stood by as Vicky swallowed each pill. The battle of the pills was over. I stayed the night with Vicky again. I spent most of the night walking the floors of the hospital to ease the stress. There were so many rooms filled with kids with cancer. I wanted to know how the other parents dealt with the stress. The stress was so intense that I had to take the day off from work.

Physical Therapy started Wednesday morning. Mike told Vicky about a carnival for the kids in the afternoon. The kids would have an opportunity to throw pies at the workers. Vicky tried several times to throw a pie into Mike's face at the carnival. Finally she asked the nurse to roll the wheel chair closer. Vicky reached forward, and rubbed the pie into Mike's face. The laughter was great therapy for Vicky. Windle and Stacy were allowed to participate in the carnival activities. Windle won a truck, Stacy won a stuffed dog, and Vicky won a large teddy bear. Vicky went to x-ray after the Carnival. The chest x-rays looked good, and indicated that the antibiotics were still working. A CT scan was scheduled for Monday. One unit of platelets was transfused after Vicky returned to he room.

Thursday morning Vicky tried to get to the bathroom by herself, but she didn't make it. She had diarrhea, which required the nurses to give Vicky a bed bath. When Vicky used the bathroom later in the morning, she failed to wash her hands. This violated two of the three rules for VRE isolation. Vicky was confined to her room. Feeding by IV was increased because Vicky was still not eating.

Gregg Adams stopped by Friday afternoon to speak with Vanessa and I. Vicky survived the lung biopsy, and no cancer was detected. Vicky came into the hospital as a 15 year-old teen. She would leave the hospital as a 17 year-old adult. However, the staff was still treating Vicky like a patient. Vicky needed to change from a patient and child into an adult. The skills needed to be a full grown female needed to be instilled into Vicky. Gregg would ask home health to start giving Vicky her baths at home. This was needed to push Vicky beyond SASSY. A 16 year-old SASSY patient is one thing, but a 17 year-old adult is all together different.

Vicky woke up Saturday morning with severe pain below her lungs. On a scale of 1 to 10, this was a ten. Tears flowed like water as she begged the nurse for pain medication. Windle and Stacy played in Vicky's room instead of the playroom because of concerns about VRE. Vicky wanted Windle and Stacy to be quiet so she could rest. Vicky was still isolated to her room, and she wanted to work on crafts in the teen playroom. She did not want to stay isolated in her room. Vicky wanted someone to help her pout, but no one would.

I took the kids to church at Ferndale Assembly of God Sunday morning while Vanessa stayed with Vicky. Vicky was given permission to go to the cafeteria with the family for lunch since her diarrhea had ended, and she was washing her hands. Vicky picked out pickles, olives, gummy bears, corn on the cob, and ice cream. The only thing Vicky ate was the corn.

Vanessa and Windle had appointments with their doctors in Fort Smith Monday morning. Windle's checkup was great. Vanessa's blood sugar was high, and she had a bacteria and fungal infection. We wondered if Vanessa and Vicky's infections were related. Vicky's CT scan was completed when Vanessa and I returned to Little Rock. The thickening on the outside of the left lung was better, but it was still there. Many of the masses were gone. Some small masses (half the size of a small fingernail) did not change; they were no smaller and no larger. A follow-up CT scan was scheduled in two weeks. If the small masses were still present, a needle biopsy on one of the masses would be performed. Dr. Stine started the process for checking Vicky out of the hospital.

The company that provided IV feeds arrived at the apartment an hour after Vicky was released from the hospital. 128 milliliters of lipids and 2 liters of TPN would run over 16 hours. All of the equipment was connected and running just before midnight. Vicky needed help pushing the IV pole when she went to the bathroom during the night. I was very tired when I went to work Tuesday morning.

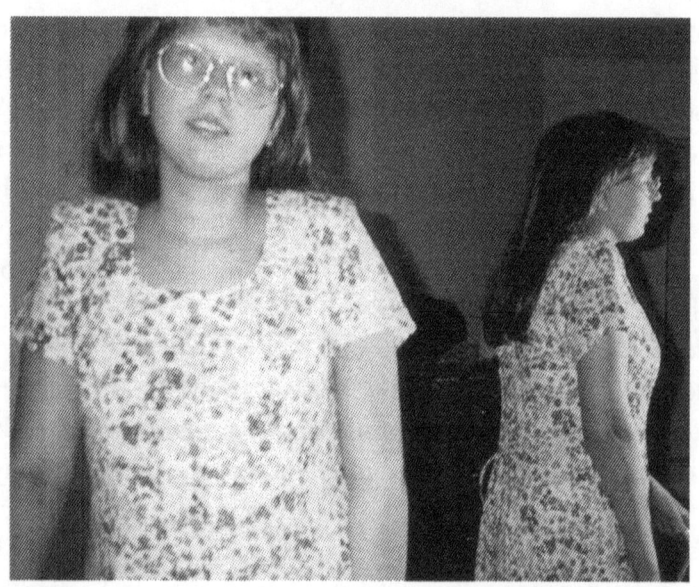

Vicky showing off her long wig in the mirror.

THE RED DRESS

"Assurance"
Real optimism is aware of problems but recognizes the solutions, knows about difficulties but believes they can be overcome, sees the negatives but accentuates the positives, is exposed to the worst but expects the best, has reason to complain but chooses to smile.

William Arthur Ward

I drove to work Tuesday, March 25, with Jamaliah, a coworker who lived in Little Rock. The one hundred-mile ride seemed to take much longer than usual on this morning. After thirty minutes at work, I had every sign of a heart attach. There was the feeling of suffocation. My hands started shaking, and paper work on the desk did not make any sense. Sweat started to flow, and a sense of passing out overwhelmed me. My left shoulder ached with pain. I walked around my office to cause the thought of passing out to subside, but the feeling only got worse. Instead of calling for help, I headed out the door. The hallway looked so long. I could hear every breath while the pain in my shoulder intensified with each step. I somehow made it to the medical office where I was placed on a bed. My blood pressure was elevated, and an EKG showed a lack of oxygen. Fluids and oxygen were started. The ambulance was called. At the emergency room a chest x-ray and follow-up EKG were normal. Medication for stress was administered, and soon I was feeling much better. I was placed on one week of leave. Burl Neal drove me back to the apartment in Little Rock.

I arrived at the apartment in time to find the home health nurse disconnecting Vicky's IVs. I laid down for a nap. I woke ten hours later when home health arrived later in the day to reconnect Vicky's IVs. The "Y" connector on Vicky's IV pole started leaking an hour after the fluids were started. I replaced the connector. The stress was manageable with my new medication and rest.

Elizabeth, Vicky's home health supervisor, came to the apartment Wednesday morning to disconnect Vicky's IVs. Vicky took a long time to get her pills swallowed. Vicky walked into the kitchen with several of her pills, and returned without any of them. I knew what happened. I checked the trash can and found Vicky's pills. Reluctantly Vicky took all of her pills. Vicky asked to go shopping at University Mall as a reward for having swallowed all of her pills. Vicky walked up the stairs to the car. I would have taken Vicky shopping even is she did not take her pills, and Vicky knew that.

Barbara is one of the technical aids on the cancer wing of Arkansas Children's hospital. Barbara told Vicky about a sale on pajamas at J.C. Penney. Vicky found a green pair of silk pajamas with long pants and a long sleeve top. Vicky then stopped to look at the dresses. The prom dresses caught Vicky's attention. I pushed Vicky in her wheel chair around one set of dresses at least five times.

Vicky pulled down a long black dress covered in sequins. Vanessa and Vicky took the dress into the dressing area. A man stood close to me while Vicky was trying on the dress. He asked a few questions about Vicky and her cancer. There was nothing unusual about the man. He wore faded blue jeans and a short-sleeved sport shirt. Vanessa soon came out of the dressing area with the black dress. It was too big. The only dress of the right size was a long red one. It was spectacular in brilliance and glitter. Vicky soon walked out to show off the red dress. Vicky had her red wig on. The dress with the wig took everyone's breath away. Vicky was absolutely beautiful in the dress. Vicky asked if I would buy the dress.

I looked at the price tag on the dress. It was much more than what I could afford. I asked if there was a layaway plan. Just then I was tapped on the shoulder. The man with the questions about Vicky asked if he could buy the dress. He said that he and his wife were saving money for such a time as this. The man paid in cash. I asked the man if he would give an address to send Vicky's journals to. The man wrote down an address and then turned to walk away. He had another dress in his hand, but no one ever saw his wife. Vanessa and I called out to thank the man, but he was gone—vanished! Vicky quickly stated that he was simply an angel taking care of her. She had her dress in her lap with a smile from ear to ear. Vicky could hardly wait to tell everyone about the dress her angel bought.

Eunice Galloway came to the apartment to visit with Vicky and Vanessa. Vicky was quick to show off her dress and tell the story about the angel. Eunice left several CDs for Vicky to listen to during the day. Eunice Galloway wanted to help so many people after the recent loss of her daughter, Laura, to cancer.

On Thursday, March 27, Vicky's feet started swelling. I called Kyla, Vicky's favorite home health nurse, and asked what to do. Kyla told me to elevate Vicky's feet, and that worked. But, there was still noticeable swelling around the ankles. The results of Vicky's blood tests indicated the need for red blood and platelet transfusions on Monday.

I arrived home with a 386 SX laptop computer and portable printer I purchased from the surplus store at work. Vicky started right in with her homework on the computer. My dad and his wife (Grandpa and Grandma) arrived in Little Rock late in the evening. My mom died several years earlier and my dad remarried. My dad and I arranged to have breakfast together in the morning.

Kyla, with home health, came to the apartment Friday morning. Vicky treated Kyla to several crazy antics, so Kyla nicked name Vicky: "Fuzzy Nut." Vicky's hair was starting to grow, and it did look very fuzzy. Vicky pinched me when I called her a "Fuzzy Nut." Vicky said that

Kyla was the only person allowed using that nickname. "Sassy" was the nickname everyone else had to use. Vicky had that "Taz" look in her eyes that said she meant it.

I went to Terry Elementary School in Little Rock for a parent-teacher conference concerning Windle. Windle was doing real good, and was coming out of his bashfulness. I then met my dad at the motel for breakfast. I rode with Grandpa and Grandma to the apartment.

After a long visit, everyone wanted to go out for Mexican food. Vicky had a ball visiting with Grandma, and Stacy took to Grandpa like a duck to water. Vanessa, Grandpa, Grandma, and I visited for a time while the 3 kids played in the arcade room. Vicky arrived back at the apartment just in time to have her IVs hooked up. Vicky received an Easter basket in the mail from one of the Assembly of God Missionette groups. She opened it in front of Grandpa and Grandma.

Grandma and Vicky visited on the couch for several hours. Vicky opened up to Grandma so naturally and adult-like. Stacy and Grandpa played and played. Windle was wound up tight and watched television to calm down. Vicky showed off her red dress and told the story of her angel.

I drove back to the motel with Grandpa and Grandma at the end of the day. The three of us went to dinner, and then visited in the motel lobby until nearly 10:00. Back at the apartment the three kids made Easter gifts for Grandpa and Grandma. When I arrived back at the apartment, Vicky sent me to the grocery store. She wanted cream cheese and black olives to snack on.

Vicky woke everyone up Saturday morning once the home health nurse disconnected the IVs. Vicky and Grandma had made plans to go shopping at the University Mall. Vicky wore her black Easter dress. It was tight on her because of what appeared to be fluid buildup. The first thing Vicky wanted to do at the mall was eat. She asked to eat at the cafeteria where she could find many different foods to choose from, but all Vicky did was nibble on a few items. Grandpa, Grandma, and I talked about taking Vicky out to eat. I told them that Vicky would always try to eat something when we took her out to eat. Vicky would also try to eat if we went to the store for a special order. I tried to explain how this always prompted Vicky to try. I told them that I was willing to do what ever it took to keep "Sassy" alive. Going shopping was another great way to keep Vicky going. Grandpa and Grandma then praised Vicky for what she did eat and encouraged her to try some more.

The Easter Bunny was at the mall. Vicky wanted a picture of her and Grandpa with the bunny rabbit. All three kids then had their picture with the bunny to give to Grandpa and Grandma. Grandma pushed Vicky's wheel chair from store to store. Vicky found a pair of shoes that matched her red dress. Grandma gave Vicky the money for the shoes. Grandma then bought a large stuffed bunny rabbit for Stacy. I had to take the rabbit to the car without Stacy seeing it. Grandpa and Grandma went back to the motel after dropping everyone off at the apartment. Terry drove to the apartment after he got off work.

The home health nurse connected Vicky to the IVs in the evening. The nurse could not find a pulse in Vicky's feet because of the swelling. Vicky promised to put her feet up. But as soon as the nurse left Vicky stated dying Easter eggs with Windle and Stacy. Terry and I went to dinner with Grandpa and Grandma. At dinner, Grandpa gave Terry $25.00 for Easter. My dad then gave me $200.00 for the family to use as needed. Terry spent the evening talking with Grandpa and Grandma. It was a wonderful time together.

Vicky was the first one up Easter morning. She woke up Windle, Terry, and me. Stacy was taken back by the large Easter bunny sitting in the chair. Vicky was excited all morning long. Vicky put on her new black dress. It looked really good on her, especially with her blond wig.

The family went to the Ferndale Assembly of God church in Little Rock Easter morning. The congregation was excited to see the whole family together. Terry met a girl who was a student at his college. She invited Terry to Chi Alpha meetings with her. Vicky was able to meet Tabitha for the first time. Vicky was able to meet several of the people who wrote to her. Vicky was so excited about being in church again. Vicky went to children's church with Stacy, and helped teach the lesson. The second, and final, part of the angel's promise to Vicky came true. Vicky stated that she wanted to start teaching in church again.

The kids participated in the egg hunt after church. Stacy only found one egg, but it was a prize egg. Windle also found a prize egg in his hunting area. The church gave away teddy bears for prizes. The church also gave Vicky a special teddy bear.

Grandpa and Grandma arrived at the apartment in time to watch Vicky get connected to the IVs again. Vanessa and Grandma went shopping to find some cards to play games. They returned with a set of Skip-Bo cards. Windle played in a manner to keep Grandma from winning. His strategy worked, and Grandma kept teasing him. Windle could not stop from laughing. Later in the evening Vicky's left stomach muscle started hurting. Big tears welled up in her eyes, and she went to bed crying. My dad said that he did not know how we were able to keep going.

Vicky asked for hugs from Grandpa and Grandma before they left. Grandpa and Grandma were headed back to California in the morning. Vicky told them that she had the most wonderful time of her life. I went to dinner with Grandpa and Grandma.

Vicky's port needle fell out during the night. I called home health to come help. I felt comfortable doing many of Vicky's procedures. But, I could not bring myself to push the port needle into a port that was buried beneath the skin. Elizabeth was on call. I warmed a jell pack to place on Vicky's sore stomach muscle. It helped the pain go away.

Terry and Windle went to school Monday morning, and Vicky went to the hospital for transfusions. Vicky weighed in at 116.1 pounds, which was a 10-pound gain in one week. Carol Godfrey was called about Vicky's weight gain and swelling. I started to get a bad headache around noon, and I took aspirin. I went to the apartment to pick up Windle after school. My headache was getting worse, so I took medication for stress and took a nap. My headache continued to get worse. I picked up Vicky when her transfusions were completed. Vicky asked to stop at Kentucky Fried Chicken for dinner. My headache was so bad I had to lie in the car while the rest of the family ate dinner. I could not stand the pain to drive home, so Vanessa drove to the apartment. It took me several minutes to gain enough strength to make it to the bed in the apartment. My pain was so intense that I could no longer lay still. I was worried that this was an aneurysm. A call was placed to 911, and an ambulance arrived just has the home health nurse arrived to connect Vicky to her IVs. I went to the Baptist hospital emergency room. Back at the apartment Vicky's temperature spiked to 101 degrees. Another ambulance was called to take Vicky to Children's hospital. Kyla and Vanessa went with Vicky.

I was checked with a CT scan. A stronger form of stress medication was prescribed. The nurse told me that I had to learn to handle the stress. I was released from the hospital. Vanessa was called at Children's Hospital to pick me up. Vicky's fever returned to normal, and she was sent back to the apartment with the home health nurse. Through all of confusion of the evening, Vicky's injection was missed.

A home health worker arrived the morning of April first to give Vicky her bath. The woman helped Vicky with her bath, helped her get dressed, and made sure Vicky had breakfast. Vicky liked this new arrangement, and so did Vanessa. I stayed home from work and took my prescribed medications for stress. Vicky made out a grocery list: Ice cream drumsticks, beef raviolis, pork and beans, baked beans, and corn on the cob. Vanessa and I spent the day at the apartment. Vicky was connected to her IV pole and went to bed. Vicky required help pushing her IV pole several times during the night to get to the bathroom.

I went back to work on Wednesday, April 2. Jamaliah, my co-worker, drove. The company doctor released me back to work, but I had to change the medication prescribed by Baptist hospital. The paperwork on my desk was late. I wrote a letter to my manager describing the difficulties returning to work following the events of Vicky's lung biopsy.

I was glad that Jamaliah drove because I could not stay awake for the ride home.

When I arrived at the apartment, Vanessa asked if the two of us could go out for dinner. Vicky said that she felt good enough to stay by herself for an hour. Windle said that he wanted to go also and got mad. Windle was disciplined, and Vanessa said she was in no mood now to go out for dinner. Vanessa went to bed and told me to get dinner at Wendy's. Vicky refused to eat anything from Wendy's and asked me to go back to Kentucky Fried Chicken for corn on the cob and baked beans. After everyone had his or her dinner I walked up to the pool to relieve the stress. The view from the pool out over the suburbs of Little Rock was breath taking and soothing. I sat there for several hours.

I drove to work by myself Thursday morning. The ride was very long again. I made two stops along the way to take short walks to stay awake. The walks also removed much of the stress in my shoulder. Terry met me at work for lunch. Terry brought all of the mail. The trip back to Little Rock was a lot easier.

I had a stress test Friday morning. Everything looked great. The stress really was the culprit. The home health nurse identified congestion in the top part of Vicky's lungs when the IVs were disconnected in the morning. The congestion was gone when the IVs were started in the evening. Vicky was very energetic, and wanted to eat more beans and corn. Vicky was up several times during the night to use the bathroom. Each time she said that she was feeling great.

Everyone was sleeping when the home health nurse arrived Saturday morning. The nurse quickly called me when she realized Vicky was in trouble. Her fever was 102.4, her blood pressure was low at 90 over 40, her respiration was 39, and her heart rate was high at 144. This reminded everyone how quickly a child with cancer could get sick. It only took me fifteen minutes to drive Vicky to the emergency room at Arkansas Children's hospital. Vicky's lungs were clear, but she had a runny nose and watery eyes. One liter of fluids was pushed and an antibiotic was started. A chest x-ray was ordered. All of the rooms on the cancer wing were full. Vicky was placed in a room on the Blue wing, but her assigned nurse worked on the Orange wing.

Vicky weighed 116.6 pounds Sunday morning. Her temperature was back to normal. The blood cultures showed a gram-positive cluster. This was indicative of a skin contamination entering the blood. Vicky's breakfast came to the Orange wing. It was not served since she was on the Blue wing. I was checking on Vicky's breakfast when the pediatrician checked her records. He stated that the team was considering the antibiotic vancomycin for Vicky's infection. I got upset when I heard the word "vancomycin." All of the troubles at church with VRE were still very painful for the family. Everything was quickly corrected, and vancomycin was not used.

Vicky transferred to the cancer ward after several rooms opened up. Vicky's port needle was replaced because it was in use for a week. There was a possibility that the infection came from the site of the needle especially since the needle fell out during the week. Doctor Becton stopped by for evening rounds. He was in the meeting that reviewed all of Vicky's lung biopsy results. It was known for sure that no cancer cells were identified. No other information was known about the tissue removed from the lung other than it did look infected. The x-ray from the previous day looked good, but did show the need for continued healing in the lung. Doctor Becton would discuss adding an amino acid to the IV feeds. A CT scan was scheduled for Wednesday.

I took Stacy to day care Monday after I put Windle on the school bus at the apartment. I had an appointment with my psychiatrist. Doctor Sunderman told me that my two episodes were called "panic attacks." He told me that most people would do just about anything to keep from having another attack. I was more than happy to take medication to keep from having another attack. Two teen volunteers helped Vicky play games on her new computer. The technician, Barbara, gave Vicky her bath and helped her get dressed into her new pajamas. Barbara and

Vicky talked about the sale at the mall, and the man who bought the red dress. Vicky asked Vanessa and I to go home so she could stay by herself during the night.

I put in a full day at work Tuesday. Vicky was released from the hospital after one unit of platelets was transfused. The amino acid called "cysteine" was added to the IVs. The IVs were connected for twelve hours instead of sixteen hours a day. The medical supply company was so impressed with the way I connected Vicky's IV's that they invited three nurses to learn how to "spike" the bottles and connect everything. I called about writing Vicky's book. One publishing company told me that there was a need for a teenage perspective on cancer treatment and survival. Vicky called Sister Sheila at 10:00 p.m. to talk about adult girl issues and the book.

I disconnected Vicky from the IV feeds Wednesday morning. On the way to the clinic Vicky asked for hash browns from McDonalds, but she did not eat any of it. I turned the car in for repairs, and then returned to the clinic in the courtesy car. I noticed that I still had the keys to the car with me. I made a quick trip to the auto shop. I made it back in time for the CT scan. When the car was finished the bill was nearly $400.00. I knew that reliable transportation was an absolute need.

The CT scan looked better, but there was still the need for healing. Most of the lesions were gone, and the lining was getting better. Cysteine was added to the IVs to aid healing. Cysteine is an amino acid that normally comes into the body through the proteins we eat. But, Vicky was not eating like a normal person. The body does not produce this amino acid. Adding the amino acid to the IVs prevented muscle mass loss, and promoted healing.

Radiation was now considered completed with the last five exposures cancelled. The last round of chemotherapy had to be administered. Doctor Stine stated that data two years after chemotherapy does not support skipping the last round of chemotherapy. If Vicky's white cell count was high enough on Monday, she would get her last round of chemotherapy on Wednesday. Vicky was excited about having an "end-of-chemo party" with Rhonda and Janet. Vicky walked to the cancer ward and visited with Rhonda. Vicky asked to eat lunch at Pizza Hut. She ate a small amount of spaghetti. Vicky asked to eat dinner at Western Sizzlin. She filled her plate with a little of everything, but ate a very small amount.

Vicky's port would flush, but it would not draw back any blood Thursday morning. The home health nurse took blood from Vicky's arm. Vicky called me at work, and asked me to bring home spaghetti without meat from Pizza Hut. During the evening the IV pumps alarmed because of low flow. The port needle was pulling out because of the weight of the tubing. The last thing Vicky wanted was another infection because of the port needle falling out. I taped the tubing, and the needle stayed where it belonged.

I stayed home from work Friday. Kyla disconnected Vicky's IV pumps in the morning. I then went to Arkansas Children's hospital to pick up a box of Vicky's GCSF. This was the injection used to increase the white blood count. I also picked up a box of large clear wound covers. They were used to keep the port needle area clean, and keep the needle from pulling out like it did. I checked on Vicky's blood counts, and made arrangements for Vicky to transfuse blood and platelets Monday morning. Carol Godfrey made an appointment for Wednesday to determine whether chemotherapy could be started. Vicky asked to eat at Chuck-E-Cheese for lunch. Her friend, who survived cancer, was no longer working there. Vicky played the games, and won over 800 tickets. She was having a great time. Vicky needed the use of an inhaler during the day because of diminished lower-left lung activity. Vicky and Windle used the evening to clean up the apartment. Vicky slept with Mom, and I slept in Vicky's bed. I got the rest I needed.

Elizabeth came to the apartment Saturday morning to disconnect Vicky's IVs. Vicky asked me if I would take her and Stacy out for breakfast at Denny's. Vicky managed to eat a few seasoned fries. I had to change a flat tire on the car. Vicky looked for cloths at Wal Mart while I had the tire repaired. Vicky then asked to eat lunch at Pizza Hut. She ate most of her spaghetti without meat. Vicky then finished her homework on her computer. I asked Vicky why I wasn't getting as many "butterfly kisses" as I used to. She said that it was because she was growing up into a woman.

Vicky used her inhaler several times Saturday. She started coughing up more clear fluids from her lungs. The inhaler showed a ten percent increase in lung capacity. Vicky kept her left arm pulled up to her chest because of the lung biopsy. The physical therapist warned Vicky that she needed to let the arm hang down to her side. As a result, Vicky's left arm was tight and swollen. She complained of the pain, and asked for Tylenol and the heating pad. Vicky pulled a muscle in her right shoulder when getting off the couch because she was not using the left arm. Vicky asked for another heating pad for her right shoulder. Vanessa said that her legs were hurting again.

Vanessa and Vicky were too tired to go to church Sunday morning. Vicky sent one of her books to church with me to give to Tabitha. Vicky asked me to pick up spaghetti without meat on the way home from church. Vicky asked for a bath after I returned from church. She said that she was tired of bed baths. Vicky asked me to obtain permission for home health to start giving her a bath again. Vicky continued to use her inhaler during the day and night.

Vicky was very tired when she was disconnected from the IVs Monday morning. Vicky arrived at the hospital, and needed three units of red blood and one unit of platelets. Vicky's white blood count was high enough to stop her injections. Vicky weighed 122 pounds. Doctor Stine said that Vicky would have chemotherapy on Wednesday. Elizabeth, with child life, was contacted to schedule an "end-of-chemo party."

Vicky checked the mail when she returned to the apartment. In the mail was her first graduation gift. Vicky asked to eat dinner at Pizza Hut. She ate two slices of pepperoni pizza along with her spaghetti.

Vanessa got mad when she asked to shop at Wal Mart and was told no. Vicky needed to be at the apartment in thirty minutes to connect to the IVs. Vanessa said that she refused to do anything anyone told her to do anymore. And, she did not care if Vicky ever got connected to the IVs. I discovered that Vanessa did not take her blood pressure medication or insulin for the past three days. I knew how the stress effected me, but Vanessa was not willing to seek help for her stress.

I called channel 5 news in Fort Smith about Vicky's "end-of-chemo party." They did not want to cover the story. Vicky called Elizabeth, with child life, and asked her to notify Rose, Sabrina, and Doctor Nicholas about the party. Rose and Sabrina were Vicky's friends in the cafeteria. The last of the IVs were connected. Vicky was excited about making it to the end of her treatment. She managed to beat the cancer. Vicky started focusing on the prom and graduating from high school.

END-OF-CHEMO PARTY

I disconnected Vicky from her IV pole Wednesday morning. Vicky dressed up in her pink dress for her "end-of-chemo" party. She was getting very excited as the nurses helped with nails and makeup. Vicky checked into the hospital weighing 124 pounds. The feeding by IVs was stopped because of the weight gain and good blood test results. Vicky asked me order spaghetti without meat from Pizza Hut for her lunch. Vicky handed out gifts to Carol Godfrey, Janet, and Rhonda. Janet was Vicky's nurse for the day. Vicky found out that her "end-of-chemo" party was scheduled for Thursday. When she was asked what she wanted to eat for her party, Vicky asked for pizza and spaghetti without meat from Pizza Hut. Vicky then asked me for more spaghetti from Pizza Hut for dinner. I visited with Gregg Adams during the evening to talk about the stress Vanessa and I was dealing with. Vicky's chemotherapy was started.

I went to Windle's school for his progress report and then back to the hospital for Vicky's party. The party was video taped by channel 11 for use in the Children's Miracle Network Telethon at the end of the month. I was interviewed. Kara Travis came to Vicky's party. Kara presented Vicky with a pink teddy bear. Kara told Vicky that she wanted the two of them to get together for glamour photos.

Vicky did not eat any of the spaghetti at her party because it had meat in it. Vicky would not smile while she was opening her gifts provided by the hospital. When I touched Vicky on the head, she turned around and bit my hand. Vicky went back to her room after the party to take a nap. Her noon pills were still by the bed. When the nurse brought in the afternoon pills, Vicky snapped at the nurse and me. Word quickly spread through the hospital that Vicky was in a bad mood. The only thing different from the day before was chemotherapy and it radically changed Vicky's mood. Vanessa and I went to the apartment. The Hip Police had a heart to heart talk with Vicky, and made her apologize for her bad attitude. Vicky called me and apologized for biting and snapping at me. She then asked for some spaghetti without meat from Pizza Hut. I took it to her, and Vicky stayed the night by herself. The night nurses continued to talk to Vicky about her bad mood during the day.

Vicky paged me at work Friday, and asked me to bring some spaghetti without meat from Pizza Hut. Vicky was being discharged when I arrived with the spaghetti. On the way to the apartment, Vicky asked to stop at Pizza Hut for fresh spaghetti. The spaghetti I brought went to the apartment. Vicky wanted to know if she could go to Branson since she missed out on the graduation trip with her school. I made reservations after giving Vicky her night pills. She went to the kitchen for a drink and quickly returned. I knew what happened. The pills were wrapped in Kleenex in the trash. I made Vicky take her pills.

Vicky was so excited Saturday morning as she made everyone hurry to the car. The motel in Branson had a heated pool, and Vicky went swimming. Vicky wanted to stay in the pool all night, but the family had reservations for the Osmond's show. The kids loved the show. Vicky asked to have her picture taken with the Osmond's, and she obtained their autographs. Stacy fell asleep on the way back to the motel. Vicky and Windle fell asleep as soon as their heads hit their pillows. Vanessa and I talked about the large swings in Vicky's mood. We questioned if Vicky was able to control her mood or if the chemotherapy controlled her mood. We knew the answer. Vicky was always "Sassy" when she felt good. Vanessa and I purposed to do all we could to help lift the spirits of kids with cancer and other life threatening illnesses and injuries. But, for now that idea would have to wait until Vicky was beyond her cancer.

Everyone slept in Sunday morning. Vicky ate watermelon for breakfast and then asked to go shopping. Vicky found writing pens that look like syringes for all of her nurses. Then she found a `57 Chevy car hat for Terry. She also bought a T-shirt and cookies for Kara. I took the cookies and T-shirt to Kara at the hospital after getting back to Little Rock.

I met Terry for lunch Monday. I gave Terry the hat Vicky bought for him. Vicky gave Kyla one of the syringe pins when her blood was collected. I called to check on Vicky's blood levels. She was scheduled for platelets and Vincristine chemotherapy on Wednesday. Vicky put on her bathing suit and helped me wash the car in the evening. I watched Vicky wash the car and thought about the lung biopsy. Vicky was supposed to be dead, but she was washing the car like she owned it. Maybe it was because Vicky owned life itself that she was so happy. Vicky checked the mail where she found $50.00 for graduation from her uncle. She asked to go to Wal-Mart to buy some cloths. Vicky asked to eat dinner at Pizza Hut. At Pizza Hut, Vicky gave the waitress a picture of her eating spaghetti in the hospital.

Vanessa and Vicky went to Pizza Hut for lunch on Tuesday, April 22. Vicky ate part of her spaghetti and took the rest to the apartment for dinner. Vicky went to the kitchen to take her evening pills, but she put part of them into the trash. When I confronted Vicky about her pills, she said that since chemotherapy was over her pills should be also. Vicky said that she was tired of taking so many pills every day. I reminded Vicky that she had one more boost of her last round of chemotherapy left on Wednesday. Vicky finally agreed to take all of her pills.

Vanessa and Vicky went to clinic 3 for her blood test and chemotherapy boost Wednesday morning. The results showed that Vicky needed 2 units of red blood and 2 units of platelets. Vicky went to day medicine for the four transfusions. Vanessa made Vicky walk from clinic 3 to day medicine for exercise. Vicky wanted to be pushed in the wheel chair. When

Vicky got back to the apartment she paged me at work to complain about having to walk. I told Vicky that the walk was good for her. When the physical therapist arrived at the apartment, Vicky was still in a bad mood. Vicky went to bed as soon as the therapist left. Half of her afternoon pills and all of her evening pills were on the kitchen counter. I made Vicky take her pills, but they came right back up within thirty minutes.

Vanessa paged me at work Thursday morning to complain about Vicky not taking her pills. Vicky was lying on the couch and was inactive. I asked Vanessa to take Vicky's temperature. Since Vicky received blood the day before she should be active. Only a fever or low blood counts takes Vicky's energy away. I went with Terry to turn in his car for a tune up. Instead of a tune up, his car needed a complete valve job. Vanessa called me as I was leaving from work. Vicky's temperature was 101.4 degrees. I called the hospital, and Vicky was given orders for a direct-admit to the 3 Gold floor. This was the first time Vicky was ever directly admitted for a fever. When I arrived at the apartment Vicky asked to have the feed tube inserted because she was having trouble swallowing to take her pills. Vicky knew that the hospital would maker her swallow her pills until a doctor gave orders to put in the feed tube. Vicky's eyes were wide and penetrating while I inserted the feed tube. There was a look of desperate need in her eyes. I knew that Sassy was hurting deep inside. This is the kind of hurt no one wants to talk about. It is a kind of hurt that is very difficult to relate to unless you have personally been there. Vicky asked to stay the night in the hospital by herself. Vanessa and I got some much-needed sleep. Each time Vicky's medications were put down the feed tube, Vicky erupted with nausea. The doctor said that this was caused by chemotherapy toxicity. Large doses of anti nausea medication were needed, which put Vicky to sleep.

Vicky's fever spiked twice during the night, and it was brought down with Tylenol. The doctor promised to give Vicky a pass for the prom Saturday night if her blood tests were negative for an infection. The blood tests were still negative Friday night.

On Saturday, April 26 Vicky woke up feeling much worse. The thrush in her mouth was severe. Vicky's platelet count was low, and she needed a transfusion. Doctor Saylors refused to allow Vicky to attend the prom with her still running a fever. Antibiotics for fungus growth in the mouth were started right away. The same fungus that put Vicky in intensive care three times, and resulted in a lung biopsy was back. Vicky asked Vanessa and I to take pictures of her prom dress to the prom. Vicky did not feel like getting out of bed because of a fever. Vanessa and I left just before lunch, and went to the high school. Mrs. Maxwell was decorating for the prom when Vanessa and I arrived. I gave Mrs. Maxwell 35 copies of the picture of Vicky in her prom dress along with some homework. Mrs. Maxwell said that Vicky was voted the prom queen. Mrs. Maxwell then said that she would take videos of the prom, and make a copy for Vicky. The seniors were looking forward to Vicky being at the prom.

Vanessa and I accomplished as many tasks as possible in eight hours at the house before going back to Little Rock. Vicky started paging me when we were near Conway wanting to know where we were. Vicky wanted Vanessa to stay the night with her. I dropped Vanessa off at the hospital and then took Windle and Stacy to the apartment.

The kids and I slept in Sunday morning instead of going to church. I was catching up on laundry when Vicky called asking for spaghetti without meat from Pizza Hut. Vicky had the doctor remove her feed tube by the time I had the spaghetti at the hospital. Vicky refused to eat the spaghetti stating that she was burnt out on it. Vicky sent me hunting for corn on the cob, pork and beans, chips, ice cream, cookies, and sweet pickles. Vicky ate a little of everything, and took all of her medications by mouth. Vicky received another platelet transfusion. I felt the rush of the weekend catching up to me, and I took the appropriate medications for the occasion. Within an hour I was doing well. It is said that chivalry is not dead; only moved. I did not get to open a door for Vicky at the prom, but I did get to move her IV pole for her in the hospital.

Vicky needed two units of red blood Monday morning. Vicky called me at work, and asked me to bring cheese pizza from Mazzio. Vicky did not eat the pizza. Vicky then asked me to get chicken nuggets from McDonalds. She ate four of the nuggets. Vicky found out that Karen Wheaton would be at Fort Smith on Friday. Vicky wanted to wear her prom dress to the concert. The doctor told Vicky she could go if her fever was gone for over 24 hours.

Vicky asked me to stop by the house after work Tuesday to pick up her comforter from her bed. I called Karen Wheaton, and told her that Vicky was going to be at the concert Friday in her prom dress. Tina Choate from the church was in Little Rock with her school group. She called and asked Vanessa to pick her up to come visit with Vicky. The two visited for several hours. Brother Dade came in the evening to visit with Vicky. Vicky needed another unit of platelets. Her temperature spiked to 101.4 degrees.

Vicky still had a fever Wednesday morning when I left for work. Eunice Galloway obtained permission to take Vicky out on the roof. The two talked about cancer, surviving, faith, and anything else that came to mind. Vicky never knew Eunice's daughter, Laura. Eunice did her best to describe Laura to Vicky. It was great therapy for Eunice. I called to check on Vicky's blood counts. The white blood count was finally starting to increase indicating that the infection was finally going away. Vicky's port needle was changed when she got back to her room. The nurse noticed a blister with a scab near the needle site. The area was cultured for infections. The only item Vicky ate all day was the cheese in packs of cheese with crackers.

I took Vicky's homework to work with me on May 1st. Mrs. Maxwell said that the seniors were putting together a package for Vicky. Terry drove his truck to school, and on the way one of the valves dropped into the engine. His car was repaired so I drove Terry to pick up the car. The dealer lowered the price $100.00 because of all the medical bills.

Vicky's fever was gone for 24 hours Thursday afternoon. She was in the process of being discharged when I returned from work. Vanessa had the car packed for the trip home. Janet told me that Vicky gave the hospital teacher a hard time about finishing her homework. Vicky needed to finish several papers in order to graduate with her class.

Vicky asked to stop to use the bathroom on the way home. She also asked for her afternoon pills. Rather than taking the pills, Vicky put them in the trash. Vicky asked me to call Terry. She wanted to meet him at Lazy Earl's restaurant for dinner. Vicky picked through her dinner and did not eat very much. I made sure Vicky took her bedtime pills.

Vicky went to her school Friday morning to visit. Vicky refused to take her pills before going to the school. Most of the seniors were on a field trip, but Brian Harris, the prom king, was there. I took several pictures of the prom queen and king. I spoke with the counselors to verify Vicky would graduate with her class. Arrangements were made for a wheel chair at the graduation ceremony. Vicky then went shopping at Wal-Mart to buy flowers. Vicky took the flowers to the cemetery and placed them on her Aunt Sheila's grave. Vicky went home to prepare for the Karen Wheaton concert. Vicky refused to take her pills before leaving for the concert.

Vicky was absolutely beautiful in her red dress and red wig. Vicky picked out three of Karen's cassette tapes to give to Terry. Karen's manager would not take Vicky's money, and said that they were a gift from Karen. Karen took time during the concert to welcome Vicky. Karen sang Vicky's favorite song: "Promise." Karen then added Vicky's name to the "Crispy Critters" song, which talks about making it through the trials of life. The family went back stage after the concert to visit with Karen. Karen was impressed with Vicky's dress. Karen told Vicky that this concert was better than any missed prom. Karen, her manager, and all the workers prayed for Vicky. Karen then told Vicky that she knew

God was working things out. Karen turned to Vanessa and I, and told us that we needed this night also. I was excited to once again experience God's living water during these spiritually dry times. For the past month I was existing on nothing more than foundational faith, but it was enough to make it. The evening with Vicky and Karen gave Vanessa and I the boost we needed to keep on keeping on. Vicky refused to take her pills before going to bed.

I drove the family back to Little Rock Saturday morning for special programs at CARTI and Children's Hospital about kids with cancer and educational issues. I learned that Vicky's Individualized Education Plan would end when she graduated from high school. The discussion about Vicky's college future was very beneficial. Windle, Vicky, and Stacy had a great time doing arts and crafts. I attended a free skin cancer screening. I learned that I had five pre-cancerous sites on my hands and face that need to be removed. I was told to take care of Vicky first; my skin could wait. But, I added the thought of skin cancer to my bag of things to worry about.

All of the families joined together at a park for the survivor's picnic. Vicky ate and drank a little of everything. She then went about pestering her doctors and nurses. She enjoyed talking with all of the kids and parents. The workers in the child life department challenged each other to see who could put the most marshmallows into their mouths. Everyone gathered to watch. Vicky's side started hurting from laughing so much. Nan Brooks gave Vicky a graduation gift. It was a beautiful bag with her initials in it. Vicky asked to go to Wal-Mart after the picnic. She purchased a mother's day gift and a long red nightgown. Pastor Graves, from the Ferndale church, called in the evening to ask me if I would serve communion in the morning service.

Vicky wore her black formal with a long bow to church Sunday morning. Pastor Graves asked me to testify prior to serving communion. I said thank you and good-bye to the church that loved our family. It was wonderful to share communion with such good friends. The power of God moved during the communion and praise time. Vicky's Sunday school teacher asked the family to come to the front of the church. The pastor anointed Vicky with oil, and the church prayed for the whole family. After church, everyone started packing to move back home for good.

HIGH SCHOOL GRADUATION

On Monday, May 5, 1997, I contacted several organizations to discuss Vicky's future plans following graduation. I spoke with the University of the Ozarks, the area Vocational Rehabilitation director, and the State Education Transition manager. I addressed the issues of education after cancer recovery. The two leading forms of childhood cancer are leukemia and brain tumors. Treatments for these cause a great amount of learning problems for children. Other forms of cancer have the similar problems because of the effects of cancer, chemotherapy, radiation, and surgery. The older the child is at the time of treatment, the less severe the learning disabilities are. All children with cancer, and their parents, are protected under the Americans with Disabilities act.

Vicky must get well enough to take neurological and psychological exams, which must be ordered by the doctor. Then the Vocational Rehabilitation director would administer an aptitude assessment from which vocational goals would be set. Finally a needs assessment for knowledge and skills accompanied with placement planning would occur. The Vocational Rehabilitation program would then start. Funding sources would be matched against Vicky's income. When she reached age 18 only SSI would count as Vicky's income. Vicky's case would be monitored until time for an employment interview. A probationary assessment during employment would fill in any identified knowledge and skill weaknesses identified by Vicky's employer. Vicky would then become a full time employee. For now, physical therapy, occupational therapy and social adjustment were the main objectives.

Vicky talked a lot about taking a part time job as soon as possible. She wanted to go to VoTech, and learn nursing skills. It would take time, but time was on her side now.

I checked on Vicky's blood counts and spoke with Carol Godfrey about all I learned about vocational rehabilitation. Vicky's white blood count and red blood count were good, but her platelet level was at 5. Vicky was scheduled for a platelet transfusion in the morning. Carol wanted to wait for all blood counts to return to normal before doing any neurological or psychological evaluations for post high school education or training.

Vicky required two units of platelets when she arrived at the day medicine clinic Tuesday morning. Vicky's eating had picked up, but not enough. The doctor told Vicky that it was time for her to stop eating like a patient, and start eating like a survivor. Vicky asked to eat dinner at Denny's restaurant. She ate half of a banana split. Vanessa and I wondered if a banana split was a proper meal for a survivor. It did qualify as a typical snack for a teenager.

CARTI called Wednesday to invite Vicky and I on a trip to Las Vegas. I was asked to go because of the large list of Vicky's medications and the need for a wheel chair. Since I was MD qualified they needed me. MD means both Mom and Dad qualified. Vicky finished all of her homework needed to graduate. Vicky received Email from her former pastor's wife who was a missionary in Cambodia. Vicky was gaining skills using computers.

Stacy woke up sick Thursday morning. Vanessa took her to Children's hospital, and found that she had a urinary tract infection. Vanessa checked on Vicky's blood counts. Her sodium level was low which was attributed to not eating well. Vicky had to start her GCSF injections again because the white blood count stopped increasing. Vicky's hair started falling out again. Vicky was not happy at all this time about her hair falling out. She liked how straight her hair was compared to how curly it was before cancer. While I was packing the car to go home, I had another panic attack. I had to take my medication and lay down for a while before the shaky feeling and sweating stopped.

On Friday, May 9, Vicky went with Vanessa and I to the high school to close out her Individualized Education Plan. Vicky completed her requirements to graduate from high school while doing homebound schooling. Vicky turned in all of her schoolbooks, and then went around trading signatures with all of the seniors. Vicky asked to eat a hamburger for lunch at Wendy's. She barely had one bite down when it came back up. Vicky went home to clean up and rest. Later, Vicky went with me to pick up Windle's birthday present. The family went to Mazzio's Pizza for Windle's birthday party. Vicky ate one bite of cheese lasagna. Vanessa and I reminded Vicky of the need to eat like a survivor now. Vicky rolled her eyes backward and stated that she did eat.

I worked Saturday while Vicky lay in bed. She claimed that she over-did herself at school the previous day. Vicky ate one bite of orange sherbet for lunch and refused to take any of her pills. Vicky woke up Saturday night crying. She was worried about how she was feeling. I asked Vicky how a feeling was different from a physical hurt. Vicky told me that feelings are those things you think about that make your heart hurt. Physical pains don't make your heart hurt. I prayed with Vicky and then rubbed her back until she went back to sleep. I realized that I was hurting just as much as Vicky. I prayed for God to take away the pain in my heart, and then I went to sleep.

I worked Sunday while Vanessa and the kids went to church. Vicky wore her red prom dress to church. Vicky went from class to class showing off her dress, and telling the story of her angel buying the dress. Johnna Boone gave Vicky a graduation gift. Vicky argued extensively about not taking her pills the entire trip back to Little Rock. She also refused to extend her arm like the physical therapist told her to do. Vicky stated that she could not eat, she could not swallow her pills, and she did not want the feed tube put in. Vicky wanted me to call the doctor to get nutrition by IVs connected. I said no.

I checked on Vicky's blood counts Monday while I was at work. Vicky needed two units of red blood and two units of platelets on Wednesday. Vicky ate half a potted meat sandwich during the day. It took Vicky until midnight to get down all of her pills. Vanessa packed all day Tuesday for the trip home Wednesday.

Windle went to school, and then everyone else went with Vicky to Children's hospital for her transfusions. On the way to the hospital Vicky became nauseated. Vicky was use to keeping her blue bucket with her in the car. Once Vicky was in the hospital bed, I took Vanessa and Stacy home. Terry then took Vanessa and Stacy to Fort Smith for two doctor appointments. I returned to Little Rock to pick up Windle and Vicky. On the way back home, Vicky became nauseated again.

Thursday, May 15 started with a breakfast just for seniors. All of the senior girls wanted their picture taken with Vicky. The graduation rehearsal was right after lunch, and Vicky started acting like one of the seniors. Vicky practiced walking from her chair, but it was too strenuous for her. Room was made for her wheel chair, and she practiced walking across the stage with me at her side.

Vicky was in the reception room of the new high school at 7:30 p.m. getting ready with all of the other seniors. You could literally see Vicky changing roles from a patient to a senior with her friends. I pushed Vicky's wheel chair onto the gym floor, and took a seat next to her. The opening prayer gave thanks for Vicky being with her friends on graduation night. The guest speaker, Ms. Mary, started as a teacher's aid the year that Vicky's class started Kindergarten. Ms. Mary traveled down memory lane with the seniors, reminding them of the many great values they learned over the years. Ms. Mary thanked Vicky for teaching the value of Grace to everyone.

Vicky was the second senior to be called to receive her diploma. As soon as she took the first step onto the stage, her classmates gave her a standing ovation. The first thing Vicky did when she got back to her spot was to check that the diploma was really there. The closing prayer asked the Lord to continue the healing process in Vicky's life.

When all of the graduates got to the back of the gym, they threw their caps into the air. Vicky was grinning from ear to ear as her cap left her hand. Back at the reception area, the school board, and many friends greeted Vicky. Being at graduation helped Vicky start the transition back to a normal life.

Vicky did not eat anything all day Friday. When I got home from work, Vicky asked to go out to eat. Vicky had me drive past every restaurant at least twice before deciding to stop at Woodard's restaurant. Vicky picked through her food, but did not eat anything. When I got back home I checked Vicky's pills. Over half of the pills were left. Vicky refused to take the rest of her pills claiming that she was tired of vomiting.

I helped Terry work on his truck Saturday. Vicky's cousin, Paula, and Amanda Morrow came to visit with Vicky. Amanda brought her baby with her. Vicky was so excited to be an adult who had graduated from high school. Vicky asked to eat dinner at the Tastee Freeze restaurant. She ordered a taco salad, corn dog, tatter tots, and a freeze. Vicky nibbled on everything. Sister Sheila called to check on Vicky. The two talked for over an hour. Vicky ate half a potted meat sandwich before going to bed.

The family went to church Sunday morning. I was able to teach my Sunday school class for the first time in several months. Vicky spent time talking with all of her friends. The family packed up, and went back to Little Rock after church. I talked Vicky into going swimming. I made her walk all the way to the pool. Vicky, Windle, and I swam in the pool for several hours. Vicky used the buoyancy of the water as she walked lap after lap around the pool.

I checked on Vicky's blood tests Monday. Vicky's platelet level was 6, and she was scheduled for two units of platelets in the morning. The physical therapist noted that Vicky's left arm was much stronger. Vicky was feeling so good about her arm that she asked to go shopping at the

University Mall. Rather than using the wheel chair, Vicky chose to walk. Vicky found another dress.

Vicky arrived at the day medicine clinic Tuesday morning for her two units of platelets. While getting the transfusions, Vicky ate a candy bar, a cookie, and a gummy worm. The first round of follow-up tests was performed. There was a kidney function test, and chest CT scan. The heart echogram, chest x-rays, CT scan of the original tumor site, and a bone scan were scheduled for Wednesday. Vicky asked to keep her port needle in so that she would not have to be stuck again Wednesday. Vicky complained through the night that her port site was hurting every time she got up, but everything looked normal.

Vicky arrived early in the morning for the second day of follow-up tests. Vicky's weight was down to 104 pounds, which was a loss of 20 pounds in a month. Carol Godfrey presented Vicky with a bath gel set for graduation. When Vicky went for her chest x-rays, she became nauseated. Then she started crying and screaming stating that something was wrong with her port needle. The nurse looked at the needle, and it was coming out. Each time Vicky stood up the needle would come out, and then it would stab her each time she moved to sit back down. Vicky was being stabbed each time she moved. A new port needle was put in after numbing medication was applied for 45 minutes. All of the tests were finally finished, and Vicky was told to wait to speak with doctor Stine about the results.

Doctor Stine said that the bone scan showed an abnormality in the upper right arm. A follow-up x-ray of the right arm was ordered. It was abnormal also. A CT scan of the right arm was ordered. It revealed problems inside the bone. Doctor Stine provided three possibilities: this was a return of the cancer; this was a different form of cancer; or this was the same infection that was in her lungs. Vicky and doctor Stine then talked about Vicky's medications. Vicky could stop the calcium and sodium bicarbonate. All other pills must be taken. Vicky's potassium level was very low. Vicky promised to follow the doctor's orders. Vicky's white blood count was high enough to stop the GCSF injections.

Doctor Stine said that the bone scan from January 15, 1997 showed slight activity of the right arm. The activity was attributed to active use of the right arm compensating for the lack of use of the left arm. The doctor stated that he did not know if cancer was present in the arm back in January.

Doctor Stine scheduled an appointment with Doctor Nicholas for Wednesday, May 28 to discuss how the bone would be biopsied. In preparation for the biopsy of the right arm, the physical therapist would aggressively work to restore as much use of the left arm as possible.

If this was Ewing's sarcoma in the bone, then radiation could kill it out. A new form of chemotherapy that has minimal impact on the bone marrow would be considered depending on the biopsy results and involvement inside the bone. Vicky was angry that she had to go back into treatment. She remembered the pain of the lung biopsy and was fearful of the impact on her good arm. She lost her appetite and asked for the feed tube to be put in. I told her no.

Vicky was going to Las Vegas June 16-18 with the radiation institute. Doctor Stine said that Vicky needed to go. Vicky also wanted to go to a camp for kids with cancer in July. The need to look forward, but remembering to enjoy the present moment was so important. Only with God's grace could Vicky keep this in focus.

Titus 2:11-13, in the Bible, states that grace is an instructor in *living*. Grace first teaches what to renounce, that is, those desires of fallen humanity that are against God and morally reprehensible. Grace then teaches how to *live* soberly, righteously, and godly. Sober living is to live in a self-controlled manner. Righteous living is being morally pure. Godly living refers to a proper fear and reverence for God. Because of God's grace, Vicky was overcoming her fear of the upcoming biopsy and possible treatments.

Just when we thought we could move out of Little Rock, and go back home, we realized that God's grace was absolutely needed to help Vanessa and I *live* with the stress. Vicky needed continued encouragement to keep *living*.

On the way back to the apartment Vicky started laughing about how her port needle was stabbing her through the night. She wanted to keep the needle in from the day before to keep from being stuck again. Instead she wound up being stuck multiple times, and the needle still had to be replaced. Proverbs 17:22 states that a merry heart does good like a medicine. I enjoyed hearing Vicky laugh in spite of the return of cancer.

Vicky started crying during the night about the diagnosis. She asked to lay with Mom and I. Vicky said that she was feeling sad inside. Vicky asked for diet Dr. Pepper and a Popsicle every two to three hours during the night. Vanessa and I were getting very tired again.

THE DEATH OF SASSY

Vicky refused to eat and take her pills all day Thursday. When the physical therapist arrived, he started on stretching exercises for her left arm. Vicky refused to participate. She allowed the therapist to move her arms and legs wherever he wanted. I took the trash out when I got home from work. As I lifted the bag to put it in the dumpster I noticed a pile of pills in the bottom of the trash. There were over two days worth of pills thrown away. Vanessa called Sister Sheila to ask her to talk with Vicky about her attitude. Vicky and Sister Sheila talked for several hours. Vicky promised to allow me to put in the feed tube Friday if she could not take her morning pills. Vicky started on her nighttime pills, but could not finish them because of gagging. Vicky called on Vanessa and I every two to three hours during the night for a drink and a Popsicle. The need to keep Vicky healthy kept Vanessa and I up most of the night.

On May 23 Vicky wanted the feed tube put in. For the previous 10 days Vicky's appetite had diminished each day, and she had fallen way behind in her medications. Ever since the diagnosis on the 21st, Vicky did not eat at all. The medical supplier, Pharma Thera, came to the apartment and inserted the feed tube for Vicky. Feeds were started at 50cc per hour, with the rate going up by 5cc every 8 hours until 100cc per hour was reached. The family packed all of the medical supplies and went home Friday night.

On Saturday Vicky visited with three of her friends: Sister Sheila; her cousin, Paula; and Johnna. The visits made Vicky feel better about her self. Another friend, Amanda Morrow, came over in the evening to watch the video of the prom with Vicky. Vicky was complaining of pain in her right arm, and morphine was needed to control the pain. The morphine kept Vicky up most of the night.

Vicky wore her black dress with a long green bow to church Sunday. I had to drop Vicky off downstairs and walk her to her Sunday school classroom. Vicky was having a lot of trouble sitting up. I drove Vicky from the side of the church to the front of the church for the morning service. Vicky had to lie on the pew with her pillow and comforter because she was so tired. Vicky, and her friend Tina, were honored as high school graduates. I addressed the church, thanking them for all of the prayers. I reminded everyone of the need to continue to pray.

I cooked lunch, and then drove the family back to Little Rock. Vicky was scheduled to have lunch in North Little Rock on Monday with Kara. When Vicky called Kara to talk about the outing, Kara had to call it off because someone in her home was sick.

Vicky did not want to get up the morning of Memorial Day. Finally, she decided to go to the zoo. The zoo did not have wheel chairs, but they did have wagons. Vicky sat in a wagon while I pulled and Stacy pushed. After two hours at the zoo, Vicky wanted to go back to the apartment because her right arm and back were hurting and her nose started bleeding. On the way back to the apartment, I stopped at Park Plaza mall to pick up an order at J. C. Penney's for Vicky. Vicky became nauseated while waiting. I was experiencing the physical side effects of the stress, and I took my medication to stop the severe headache. Everyone took a nap after getting back to the apartment. Vicky asked to take a bubble bath in the evening. She got into the bathtub on her own, but I had to lift Vicky out because her right arm was hurting. Vicky's tongue was covered in white thrush, but she refused to scrub her tongue. She said that she was tired of throwing up. Vicky asked for a heating pad to use on her right arm when she went to bed. At 2:00 a.m. Vicky woke up because of a storm. She pushed her feed pump and climbed in bed with

Vanessa and I because she was scared of how she was feeling. Rain was falling on the window while tears were falling on Vicky's pillow.

I took Vicky to Children's hospital on the 27th for her blood test. Her counts were low. She needed two units of red blood and one unit of platelets. While Vicky received her transfusions, she sent me to Wal-Mart with $25.00 to buy her an outfit. Vicky said she was too tired to go shopping. For Vicky not to want to go shopping, something had to be wrong. I met Sheila Terrill in the hospital. Her son, Jason, was recently diagnosed with Ewing's sarcoma. Kara stopped by to visit with Vicky. Kara was being admitted for another round of chemotherapy. Vicky started feeling much stronger after her transfusions.

Vicky met with Dr. Nicholas on Wednesday to discuss the biopsy. He ordered a MRI of the right shoulder to make sure that only the bone was involved. This was the first time Vicky ever became nauseated while inside the MRI machine. Dr. Nicholas reviewed all of the test results, and scheduled surgery for Friday afternoon.

At 9:00 a.m. Thursday, I was paged by the home health nurse. When I got Vicky up in the morning she was feeling fine. But, at 8:30 Vicky had all the signs of a bad infection. She had a temperature of 102 degrees, her blood pressure was low, and her heart rate was high. Vicky was unable to walk, and an ambulance was called. Vanessa left the apartment in such a hurry that she forgot Vicky's medication list. Vanessa paged me, and had me fax a copy of the list to the doctor. Without the list, the doctor was inclined to put Vicky in intensive care. Vicky went to the oncology ward after the list of medications was received. Vicky was given an antibiotic, and her blood pressure dropped. Medication was required to control blood pressure, and Vicky's sides started hurting. As the antibiotic killed the bacteria, the bacteria released toxins into the blood stream, which caused the blood pressure to drop. There was talk once again of placing Vicky in intensive care. Doctor Becton ordered an ultrasound of the kidneys to make sure the side pain was only coming from sore muscles. Dr. Nicholas wanted to do the biopsy Friday if Vicky was stable. At 8:00 p.m. Vicky started having the shakes. Her blood pressure dropped, her heart rate increased, and her temperature spiked. I called Brother Dade to ask him to help pray, especially for the infection. Vicky's blood pressure continued to drop, and she was placed on a heart monitor. Vicky was moved to a room closer to the nurse's station. Once again Vicky was scared of dying.

The test result of Vicky's blood showed fast growing bacteria, and the third generation antibiotic, vancomycin, was started. It was not known yet if the bacteria was VRE. The results of the ultrasound indicated that the kidneys and bladder looked good with no signs of cancer. Vicky called the youth director for the Assemblies of God, and asked him to come pray with her because she was scared of dying. Brother Nordin came, and prayed with Vicky. Vicky was transfused with two units of red blood and one unit of platelets in preparation for the surgery. At the last minute the surgery was canceled because Vicky's blood pressure was out of control again.

On Saturday the infection was identified, and it was not VRE. The bacteria did require the continued use of vancomycin to kill it. Thrush started growing in Vicky's mouth, and liquid nystatin was required. Vicky said she had a puzzling dream during the night.

"She was following one set of footprints along the beach, which stopped at the edge of the ocean. The water rolled back revealing a picture of a dove with a circle around it. Suddenly the water rolled back, and the dove flew away into the sky. The Lord revealed the answer to Vicky. She was following someone who had already gone the same way she was going. Just when it seemed like the end of the road, the Lord showed her that the Spirit was leading from here on. The Spirit would take her to new heights in the Lord."

Windle and I went to the Arkansas Children's Dreams party at the Wild River Country Water Park. Over 300 people were in attendance. Ken Abbot barbecued chicken, hamburgers, brisket, and turkey. Vicki Davis was sad that Sassy could not be there. Vicki sent passes back with me to take Vicky to Wild River Country when she got better. Because of Vicki Davis' poor health, Arkansas Children's Dreams would no longer fund dreams for sick kids. I thanked Vicki Davis for filling the dream that created "Sassy." I started thinking of how I could help to bring back funding to fill the dreams of very sick kids. But, that thought would have to wait.

Vicky's nurse, Shannon, taught Vicky how to use imagery relaxation to control the pain in her sides. Vicky asked me to roll her around the outside of the hospital. Vicky enjoyed the quiet and sun. She stopped to look at the flowers. Vicky said that if God could take care of the flowers then God could take care of her.

The Children's Miracle Network telethon was televised Sunday. The story of Vicky, and an interview with me, came on around 11:30. Vanessa, Windle, Stacy, and I went to the Park Plaza Mall in the afternoon to watch the telethon. The representatives from the Clarksville Wal-Mart mentioned that Vicky was in the hospital, and said "hello" to her. Vicky was watching. At the end of the telethon, Windle and Stacy went on stage to celebrate the success of the telethon. Most of the kids were throwing confetti, but Stacy was trying to clean it up. Later in the evening Vicky asked me to take her on a stroll around the outside of the hospital again. Vicky was fascinated watching the large helicopter land. She wanted to know if the child on the helicopter might have cancer.

At midnight, Vicky was informed that she would have surgery Monday afternoon. Vicky did not sleep most of the night. Vicky's back started hurting Monday morning. She had me rub her back for several hours while using imagery relaxation to control the pain. Dr. Nicholas spoke with the pastor and me at length after the surgery. This is CANCER. The pain in Vicky's arm was from the cancer pushing outward on the bone. The mass was the size of a cigarette, and the doctor removed about 70 percent of it. Part of the tumor was dead, but part of it was alive. Vicky found out that Karen Wheaton would be in Little Rock

Friday night. The doctor said that she could go if she was stable. One of the nurses in clinic 3, Cynthia, volunteered to go with Vicky.

Vicky was told Tuesday that her incision was two inches long. A "key hole" opening to the bone was made. The bone would always be weak, and Vicky needed to protect the arm. Vicky would have a removable cast made later. Doctor Becton stated that Vicky could attend the Karen Wheaton concert and go to Las Vegas. An overall action plan would be discussed Wednesday.

Wednesday was Windle's last day of school. I stopped by the school to create his Individualized Education Plan for the next school year. Vicky started passing blood clots in her stool. One unit of platelets was transfused to control the bleeding. It was believed that the feed tube was irritating the intestinal tract, and causing bleeding. The preliminary report from the pathologist was positive for tumor cells consistent with Ewing's sarcoma. There was no evidence of any infection in the pathologist's report. Vicky's abdomen, side, and back pain was getting worse. This could be from radiation damage to the lumbar vertebrae or surrounding nerves. It could also be cancer. Nerves in this area go to the diaphragm, which was the location of Vicky's most intense pain. Touching Vicky's back made the pain worse, and relaxation exercises made the pain go away.

On Thursday Vicky became nauseated after taking her pills and threw up a large volume of fluid. Vicky asked me to change her bed while she was given a bath. Vicky was able to walk to the bathroom and use her right arm. When she returned to her bed, Vicky pulled at the tape on her nose that was holding the feed tube in place. Vicky's lungs were congested with fluid. The feed tube was irritating Vicky's nose which was causing fluids to go into her lungs. She took a deep breath and slowly pulled out the two feet of tubing from her nose. Vicky was getting pretty good at taking the feed tube out without gagging. The nurse came in to change the dressing on Vicky's right arm and noticed the feed tube was removed. Vicky said that the tube was out in order to go to the Karen Wheaton concert tomorrow. Vicky took her evening pills and became nauseated again. She asked me to give her a bath rather than telling the nurses. Vicky wanted out of the hospital in order to visit with Karen. The pain team placed Vicky on a new 12-hour slow release morphine pill in preparation to go home the next day. Vicky asked for medication for her nausea. The medications put Vicky to sleep. Every time Vicky had to take pills I would rub Vicky's back. That worked to keep the pills down. I spent the night rubbing Vicky's back and stomach. As long as I helped Vicky control the pain, her pills stayed down, and she rested. I didn't get much rest.

On Friday, June 6, Vicky was given two units of red blood for two purposes. It would help Vicky feel better when she went home, and it could cause the platelet count to come up sooner. The pain team put an electrical pulsing machine on Vicky's stomach. This worked much like me rubbing her stomach, and Vicky liked the way it took away the pain. Vicky and Gregg Adams talked at length about her diagnosis. Vicky was fully aware that she would die if the cancer in her arm was not killed, and there was a strong possibility that there were more cancer cells in her body. Vicky was scared of dying and very upset that her "Sassy" attitude had died. Dr. Stine got the full report on the biopsy, and the cancer cells had mutated themselves to be immune to standard forms of chemotherapy. Vicky was released at 1:30 p.m. She was to return Wednesday and Thursday of the following week for a full set of scans from head to toe. Vicky's clinic nurse, Cynthia, agreed to sit with Vicky at the concert.

Vicky took a nap until time to go to the Karen Wheaton concert. Vicky was hurting so much at the concert that she had to lay on the front pew. I gave Vicky some morphine, but it wasn't controlling the pain. The electrical unit was working on Vicky's stomach, I was rubbing her back, and Vicky's nurse was rubbing her feet. But, Vicky's pain continued to get worse. During the concert Karen laid hands on Vicky several times while singing songs of healing and faith. Karen held my hand while she sang, "He'll do it again." Finally at 10:00 p.m. Vicky begged to go to the emergency room. Her face was soaked in tears. The pain was more intense than the desire to be with Karen. When Karen saw Vicky leaving, she took time to give her a hug and kiss. Cynthia stayed at the concert to inform Karen of what was going on with Vicky. Cynthia called the emergency room after the concert to pass on a message to Vicky from Karen.

While laying in the emergency room, Vicky became nauseated. A light green fluid covered the bed and floor. X-rays of Vicky's abdomen showed her intestinal tract full—she was constipated. Vicky was put back in the hospital, and a new feed tube was inserted. Medications to induce a bowel movement were started. I stayed with Vicky, and Vanessa took the kids to the apartment.

Karen Wheaton said she woke up Saturday morning at 6:05 with the Spirit prompting her to go visit Vicky. Karen talked at length with Vicky, and then prayed for her. Karen told Vicky about plans to make another video, and Vicky could have a front row seat. I didn't have my medication with me, and by the time Vanessa brought it to me I was hurting so badly that the nurses were worried. I took the kids to the apartment and relaxed with them at the pool for several hours. Vanessa called me to tell me that Vicky had several open sores on her. The doctor cultured two of the sores.

I took the kids to Sunday school at the hospital. Vicky now had several more small spots on her, and Dr. Stine was very worried. Samples sent to the pathologist confirmed the worst. Vicky had chicken pox. Vicky was immediately removed from the floor, and placed in a negative pressure isolation room on the fourth floor. Vicky had bumps coming up everywhere. Vicky's white blood count was high enough that she should survive with medications. But, if her counts bottom out, the outcome would be different. Because Windle and Stacy were exposed to Vicky's chicken pox, they were not allowed to enter the hospital until the end of the incubation period of 14 days. This placed quite a hardship on the family. Only Vanessa or I could go the hospital. One of us had to stay outside of the hospital with Windle and Stacy for two weeks.

If either Windle or Stacy came down with Chicken Pox, they would both be banned from the hospital for the duration of the illness. On the weekend of May 24 and 25 Vicky went home and attended church. It was during this time that Vicky was around someone with chicken pox. Chicken pox is a virus that attaches itself to skin cells. These skin cells rub off and move through the air. These infected skin cells are breathed in. This was why Vicky was immediately moved to a negative pressure isolation room. Vicky's skin was a source of infection that could harm other kids with a weak immune system. Vanessa said that it was terrible that people at church were scared of getting VRE from Vicky and that they did not realize that Vicky could die if someone brought chicken pox to the church.

Vicky was given a morphine pump to help with her pain. Vicky's intestinal tract was not tolerating any of her feeds or medications. The pediatrician stopped all feeds and most medications for the day to allow Vicky's intestinal tract to heal. Vicky continued to swell, and x-rays of the abdomen showed complete bowel blockage. An ultrasound found stones in the gal bladder. Vicky was suffering from an acute gal bladder attack. Fluids were suctioned from Vicky's stomach, and two liters of backed up fluid were removed.

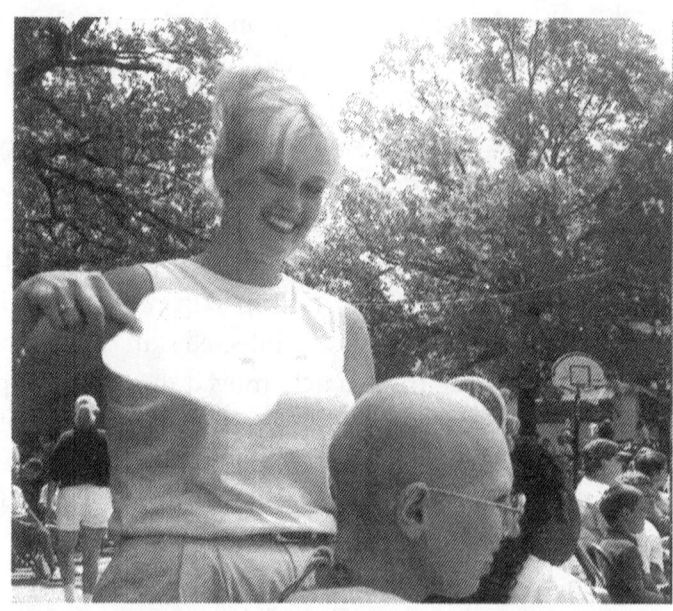

Sharon (Reier) Bergman keeps Vicky cool at Camp Barnabas.

CAMP BARNABAS

Since Windle and Stacy were exposed to Vicky's Chicken Pox, they were banned from all areas of the hospital for 14 days. The cancer wing (3rd floor) required the kids to stay away for 21 days. I took the kids to stay with a family in the church. I stayed in touch with work through Email at the hospital library.

Vicky's scans were canceled, and Vicky's trip to Las Vegas with the radiation institute was canceled because of Chicken Pox. Vicky would require radiation to the right arm for the purpose of pain control. Without radiation, the cancer would grow and break the bone at the location of the biopsy. If enough radiation were given to kill the cancer, then good bone marrow would be destroyed also. If the cancer showed up in another bone, the process of high dose radiation would continue until Vicky ran out of bone marrow. Then there would be death. What had to be found was a chemotherapy drug that would kill the remaining cells without killing the bone marrow. There was one such drug is phase one testing in Texas. Radiation was on hold until the Chicken Pox cleared up. Everything and everyone was waiting on Chicken Pox.

A bacterial infection, on top of constipation, on top of Chicken Pox, on top of a gal bladder attack, on top of surgery had Sassy down. The Chicken Pox affected the liver and intestines such that the inflamed gall bladder was causing severe swelling and pain. There was a concern that part of Vicky's pain below the diaphragm was associated with the cancer found in her right arm. Isolation for Chicken Pox prevented running any scans to verify this assumption. Dr. Stine talked to Vanessa and I about setting up hospice care at home for the short time many people thought Vicky had left. Vanessa stayed in the room with Vicky at night, and I slept in the waiting room. Three to four times each night Vicky had me called to come and talk about "things." Vicky wanted to know if she was really going to die. She wanted to know why she was selected to have cancer. She wanted to know if she could become a nurse after the cancer was cured. Vicky expected honest answers from me, and this kept me on my knees before God.

God finally answered a question I had for the past 18 months: "What will happen after Vicky is healed?" Early in 1996, I asked God if Vicky would be healed of cancer, but God did not answer this question until today. With a clearness of understanding God answered by first asking several surprising questions. When God healed the man born blind, how long did he live? When God healed the Centurion's daughter, how long did she live? When God healed the woman with the issue of blood, how long did she live? When God raised up Lazarus, how long did he live? These types of questions continued, and then God very plainly stated that His Word is silent on this issue. God said that he expects obedience to His Word, not a sacrifice in following examples of others. God said that if the life of an individual healed were laid out in His Word, people would try to follow that example rather than obey the Word. God then said, whether 15 days or 15 years, the healing belongs to God, and the number of days belongs to Him.

Vicky received a lot of mail from the staff at Camp Barnabas. They were all praying for her and looking forward to seeing her at camp on July 10th. Camp was only four weeks away, but Vicky was confident she would attend. Several women who attended the Karen Wheaton concert came to visit and pray with Vicky. A group of women from our church came to visit and pray with Vicky. A co-worker, and his family, came to visit. Vicky enjoyed visiting with each one. Vicky wanted Sister Sheila to visit. But, she could not visit with Vicky because she never had Chicken Pox.

Vicky continued to throw up large volumes of green bile. Bile is a salt created by the gal bladder and is used to digest fats. Each time Vicky ate a food with fat in it, more bile was produced.

On Tuesday, June 10 Vicky's feed tube was removed, and she started taking liquids by mouth. But, every five to ten minutes bile would uncontrollably come up. Vicky was so swollen that none of her panties fit. She gained four pounds in 24 hours. When Vicky tried to sit up she needed help because of the severe swelling. The doctor ordered another set of x-rays to look at Vicky's abdomen. There appeared to be an air aneurysm of the colon. An ultrasound was order for verification. Ultrasounds showed the bladder full, the colon full, and stones in the gal bladder. There was an apparent infection of the gal bladder. Every time the gall bladder contracted it was irritated by the stones and infection. This was the source of Vicky's pain. The large amounts of bile salts were irritating the intestinal tract, and shut it down. Vicky was ordered to have nothing by mouth for two days. IV administered all fluids and medications. Fluids were suctioned from Vicky's stomach overnight. As the fluids were removed, fluids flowed from the intestinal tract to the stomach. Then the body fluids flowed into the intestinal tract. This cycle caused Vicky's blood pressure to drop.

The discovery of stones in Vicky's gall bladder on June 8 started her on the road to recovery. With the gall bladder slowed down by medication, the swelling and pain subsided. Over two liters of fluid was removed from Vicky's stomach on the 11th. Her urine output was more than her fluid input.

On Thursday, June 12 all of Vicky's pain control was removed, including the morphine pump. Vicky started to take clear liquids, but they did not leave the stomach. After one hour all of the fluids plus more bile salts were suctioned from Vicky's stomach. The doctor said that the Chicken Pox was over, but Vicky would stay in the isolation room for now. This was to protect Vicky from picking up any secondary infections. Vicky's fever was still going up, and blood was still in the stool. Dr. Stine wanted to keep Vicky on antibiotics in case the Chicken Pox allowed a bacterial infection to set up in any of the internal organs.

Vicky started feeling better Friday. She called Rhonda to tell her that "Sassy" was back. She also told her that she believed she could become a nurse! Sassy declared vengeance on Satan for what he had tried to do to her.

Physical therapy helped Vicky exercise her legs and arms. The surgery team checked in on Vicky. They were ready just in case her gal bladder needed to be removed. I met Terry, and attended a truck and car show and swap meet. I then picked up Windle and Stacy and took them to the apartment. Vanessa and I swapped places Saturday.

Vicky was finally moved back to the cancer floor Sunday, June 15, after 7 days of isolation. Shannon, a 3rd floor cancer nurse, saw Vicky riding in her bed. Shannon asked why Vicky wasn't walking. The look on the 4th floor nurses was of surprise as Vicky smiled from ear to ear, and shouted back at Shannon. Vicky said that she was proud of the fact that she could fool those who did not know her. Shannon requested to be Vicky's nurse, and started the scheduled round of medications. Vicky did not want to take her medications and tried to call Shannon's bluff. Vicky lost, and "Sassy" declared she would get even. Shannon proved to have a stronger will than Vicky, but it made "Sassy" stronger.

Vicky tolerated a liquid diet, and was moved to a regular diet. But, McDonald's hash browns and KFC chicken caused the gall bladder to revolt. Vicky vomited large volumes of green fluid, and swelled again. The stomach tube was put back in, fluids removed, and her blood pressure dropped. After two hours of nothing by mouth, Vicky was placed on a fat-free diet. You would think that Vicky's world came to an end. The dietitian helped Vicky fill out the menu, and the only thing that Vicky could not get fat-free was peanut butter and pecan pie. Vicky's favorite was fat-free macaroni and cheese followed by fat free spaghetti. Vicky started blaming herself for eating fatty foods. Her night nurse, Sandy, let her know that this minor setback was not Vicky's fault.

Vicky was allowed to eat breakfast Monday morning in the cafeteria with Vanessa and I. On the way back to the floor Vicky found her nurse, Rhonda, on the phone. Vicky heard Rhonda tell the person on the other end of the phone that "she was working." Vicky shouted out that Rhonda has never worked a day in her life. Everyone on the floor heard it, and Rhonda was unable to fire back at Vicky. Vicky was laughing all the way back to her room. Vicky was proud of herself for getting one up on Rhonda.

CT and bone scans were completed in the evening. The bone scan showed no new sites. It did show increased activity at the site of the biopsy. Dr. Saylors and Dr. Stine discussed the need for radiation, and decided to give a dose large enough to kill the cancer. Doctor Stine told Vicky that she should go to camp Barnabas. The CT scan showed the illius (aneurysms) of the colon. This was probably caused indirectly by the Chicken Pox. As the intestines shut down the pressure inside built up, and the walls of the intestines ballooned. The CT scan also showed thickening of the lung lining near the original cancer site in the left shoulder. The doctors felt this was thickening in response to an irritant. I told Vicky that the pediatrician and radiologist were trying to locate her brain. Vicky started throwing her stuffed animals at me, and it was obvious that Vicky's right arm was very strong. Windle and Stacy were released to go anywhere in the hospital except the cancer floor. They could go on the cancer floor after Friday if they still did not show signs of Chicken Pox.

Dr. Nicholas x-rayed Vicky's right arm Wednesday, and found that the cancer was growing at an alarming rate. The bone was eaten away such that the bone could easily break. Dr. Nicholas ordered a two piece brace and recommended starting radiation right away. The material to make the brace fascinated Vicky. It is a plastic that is hard at room temperature, but easily molded when placed in hot water. Vicky made a cast for Mickey. Vanessa took Stacy to the doctor because of a fever. Stacy did not have Chicken Pox, but she did have a urinary tract infection.

During the night Vicky asked Sandy for a padded rocking chair. Vicky and Sandy talked about anything and everything most of the night. Vicky said that the two of them learned how to understand each other. Vicky could get out of the chair by herself, but she needed help getting out of bed.

Vicky and I rode Angel 3 to CARTI Thursday, June 19, for a consultation. Dr. Harris ordered 3,000 Rads over 10 days. The skin would probably burn, but that could be treated. The physical therapist started exercising Vicky's muscles when she got back to the hospital. Vicky was having trouble getting out of bed with the cast on. She needed to use the bathroom, and did not make it. She had diarrhea all over her bed. Vicky lost the privilege to leave her room again because of VRE isolation issues.

Vicky took pictures of Elizabeth and Michelle when she attended the survivor's picnic. Vicky put them on three bulletin boards in the hospital. The pictures showed the two stuffing their mouths with marshmallows. Both women vowed to get even with Vicky. Every time Vicky saw Elizabeth or Michelle she reminded them of the pictures and laughed.

Vicky rode Angel 3 again on Friday, June 20th, and then was discharged from the hospital. Vicky's list of medications was much shorter. When Vicky got back to the apartment, the women in the office gave her a T-shirt and lots of hugs. Vicky wanted to go shopping for fat-free foods at Kroger. Vicky was amazed at all of the selections available. Vicky was doing better than she had in the past two months. Everyone went swimming at the pool and stayed until the sun went down.

Vicky wanted breakfast Saturday at Denny's before going home for the weekend. She ordered an egg substitute omelet, dry hash browns, and dry toast. Vicky liked her breakfast. As soon as Vicky got home, she wanted to go to the church picnic. Vicky visited with her friends and ate a plate full of low fat snacks

On Sunday, Vicky went to her Sunday school class and then helped teach Children's church. I drove the family back to the apartment, and Vicky helped cook dinner. She ate cream corn, fat-free mashed potatoes with fat-free gravy, spaghetti, and fat-free bean dip with baked chips. Vicky, Windle, and I went to the pool for the evening.

On Monday morning, I found out that Pulaski home health had discharged Vicky because they apparently expected her to go home and die. God and Vicky chose to disappoint them! Home health refused to order physical therapy because of fear of breaking Vicky's right arm. Vicky and Vanessa went to CARTI, and Vicky walked in and out without need of her wheel chair. Windle went to church camp for the week. At my work, members of the Valley Auto Club in Russellville asked permission to hold a benefit to help with Vicky's expenses. Members of the Pope County Bass Club also asked to help with a benefit. Several of my coworkers gave the family money and gift certificates. Friends at church set up two bank accounts at home, and announced the family need on the radio. Vicky spent the evening shopping at Wal Mart.

On Tuesday Vicky went to Pizza Hut for spaghetti without meat. She really liked the spaghetti when she found out it was low in fat. The family went to Luby's cafeteria for dinner with the CARTI pals. Vicky met Jennifer, a CARTI employee close to Vicky's age. Vicky and Jennifer exchanged phone numbers. I went to the pool late in the evening to relax and get rid of a severe headache.

Vanessa took Vicky to clinic 3 Wednesday morning for blood tests. Vicky's blood test indicated that she would need two units of red blood and one unit of platelets by Monday. Vicky then went to CARTI for her radiation treatment to her arm. Before leaving, Jennifer gave Vicky a bucket full of angel gifts. My coworkers sent Vicky $200.00 in Wal Mart gift certificates. Vicky asked to go out for dinner. She ate half of a fat free cheese omelet. Everyone went to the pool after dinner. Vicky had to use the bathroom while at the pool. She walked all the way to the apartment and back to the pool while holding my hand. Her legs were getting much stronger. Vicky was excited about her renewed strength.

On Thursday, June 26, Vicky received a Pooh short set while at CARTI for the radiation treatment. Terry took a day off from work, and drove to the apartment. The family went to Wild River Country with passes provided through Arkansas Children's Dreams. Vicky stayed 6 hours, and especially enjoyed riding the rafts around the lagoon. Looking at the boys was a close second. Every minute was filled with laughter. After dinner Vicky asked to go shopping at Wal Mart with her gift certificates.

Vicky woke up early Friday morning screaming. Her eyes were filled with tears, and she had a look of panic. Her right calf muscle was in a tight knot. I had to move her foot and massager her calf before she could go back to sleep. The family went home after Vicky's treatment at CARTI. Vicky went directly to the church for an all night lock-in with her youth group. The girls stayed up all night long, and the boys' hair was coated with toothpaste when they feel asleep. Vicky slept most of the day Saturday. Saturday evening, Vicky invited her Aunt Paula and Jenny over for a fat-free Mexican dinner.

The family went to church Sunday. Vicky joined Children's church for a skating party after church. It was obvious that Vicky's blood level was low, but she pushed on because she had made plans to have dinner at Chuck E Cheese in Little Rock. Vicky and Stacy talked about all the games they were going to play while I drove to Little Rock. Vicky helped Stacy play games until Chuck E. Cheese closed. Vicky was asleep by the time she got back to the apartment.

Vicky went to day medicine Monday morning for her transfusions. She received two units of red blood and one unit of platelets. She then stopped at CARTI for her next round of radiation. Vicky called Jennifer, and asked if she would go to a movie with her. Vicky and Vanessa talked about fixing dinner before Vicky went to the show. Vanessa wanted meat in the dinner meal, but Vicky wanted hers fixed fat-free. Vanessa said she was tired of cooking fat-free meals. Vanessa went to bed and told me that I would have to fix the meals from now on. Vicky and

Jennifer went out to an evening show. Vicky was so excited to have a friend like Jennifer.

I visited my doctor Tuesday morning for a checkup on the stress. I was told that no one could make Vanessa get help for the stress. I was also told that it was all right to walk away from the stress every now and then. When Vanessa responds to the stress by walking away, I could best help by stepping in to take over. Vanessa was starting to limp because of pain in her leg, knee and hip. Vanessa and I went to dinner alone. Vicky stayed in touch with the pager and cell phone. Vicky spent the evening talking about camp Barnabas, going back to school, and getting a job.

Vicky received her last round of radiation on Wednesday, July 2nd. Vicky was excited that she was beyond cancer treatment again. It was time to start the follow up exams again. Johnson County home health nurses would draw Vicky's blood on Tuesday. The Pulaski County home health discharged Vicky to hospice care rather than to Johnson County home health. They apparently were still expecting Vicky to go home to die. Vicky was scheduled for transfusions in one week. It was time to move back home. Vicky asked to have Stacy's birthday party at Chuck E Cheese before moving home.

I took a carload of things home with me when I left for work Thursday morning. Vanessa took Stacy to Children's hospital for a follow-up appointment. Vicky took the chance to walk up to 3 Gold, and visit with Kara. Vicky remembered going through what Kara was experiencing with this round of chemotherapy. Kara was very "chemo puny." Vanessa and I took the opportunity to go to dinner alone again.

Vicky woke me up early on the 4th of July. She asked to eat breakfast at Denny's restaurant. Vicky was getting good at ordering fat-free foods at a restaurant. Vicky then went shopping for Stacy's birthday gift and a watermelon. We had fat free hot dogs and watermelon for lunch. The family spent the afternoon at the pool, and then watched fireworks. There was more to celebrate than the birth of a nation.

On Saturday, the whole family spent the morning in the pool. Vicky called Jennifer to visit with her. Jennifer and her sister, Laura, brought Vicky a box of cloths, and then the three went out to an afternoon movie. They watched "Liar Liar," and Vicky laughed more than she had in months. Vicky baked a fat-free cake for Stacy's birthday party. Vanessa and I asked Vicky how many birthday parties Stacy was going to get. Everyone just laughed.

On Sunday, July 6, the family went to church in North Little Rock where Tim and Melissa O'Brien pastor. Tim and Melissa were Vicky's youth pastors several years ago. It was so good to visit with old friends, and talk about our experiences and God's mercy. I packed the car full, and drove home. Terry and I drove back to the apartment.

On Monday, July 7, the family moved out of the apartment. Terry left early with one of the cars packed full. Vicky stopped at the apartment office, and had her picture taken with the staff. The family was given an invitation to visit at any time. When Vicky got home she pulled out her address book. She talked with anyone who would answer their phone and told them that she was home again.

Vicky packed for camp Tuesday after Johnson County home health drew her blood. Vicky was excited about going to camp. I called to check on the results of the blood tests. Vicky needed blood and platelets right away. She was scheduled to transfuse the next day. Vanessa did not want to drive to Little Rock by herself. I called Children's Medical Services (CMS) to take Vanessa and Vicky to Little Rock. There was an opening on the van.

On Wednesday, Vicky and Vanessa rode the CMS van to Children's hospital where Vicky received two units of red blood and one unit of platelets. Wednesday night, Vanessa and Vicky packed Windle's cloths for camp. Vicky asked to eat dinner at Pizza Hut. Vicky's friend, Tina, was the waitress. Vicky enjoyed talking with Tina. Both Windle and Vicky had trouble sleeping while thinking about camp.

Terry kept Stacy while the rest of the family left for camp at 8:00 A.M. Vicky and Windle arrived at Camp Barnabas, in Missouri at 2:00 p.m. They were so excited that they could not sit still for more than an hour at a time during the ride. Every hour there was a stop for a drink, a bathroom break, or both. Windle and Stacy talked the entire trip.

The rain was falling when Windle and Vicky arrived at camp. Vicky's counselor gave Vanessa and I a 30-minute tour of the camp, and the whole time Vicky never needed her wheel chair. The counselors then took Vicky and Windle to their cabins. The theme for the week of camp for kids with cancer is called "Eagles Flight." Vanessa and I headed home. The sun came out and a rainbow appeared over the hills of camp Barnabas.

What all happened at camp was amazing. Mr. Henry O. Head, known as Heno, wrote an unedited book about all the events of the week. Heno talked to many of the counselors and kids about all the events and special moments. It is best to leave those events in Heno's book. Here is an excerpt from chapter 18:

> ...On the last evening Vicky asked, "Sharon, can we get up early in the morning and go around camp. It's my favorite time of day. Everything is so soft and quiet."
>
> "Sure. It's mine, too. Let's get up at six."
>
> The next morning they woke early, dressed and slipped out of the cabin, leaving the others sleeping. Sharon wheeled Vicky along the path toward the office. Then they took a left and headed down the new asphalt road to the pool. It was a trip that would have been to rough over the rocky road in years past. Blevins' generosity was paying results.
>
> Vicky was right. It was soft and quiet. Overhead, the first hint of sunlight filtered through the canopy of leaves. On either side of the road dew sparkled and shimmered on the lush carpet of grass. Roses bloomed along a wooded fence line. Later, there

would be cabin doors squeaking and slamming, showers running, dogs barking…morning sounds. But for now, all was still.

Sharon was reminded of that hymn,

I come to the garden alone, while the dew is till on the roses…

She eased Vicky alongside the pool. There, Sharon stopped
near a bench. She sat and held Vicky's hand. For the longest time
neither spoke, just watching the mist rise from the water.

Looking toward the deep end of the pool, Vicky broke the
silence. "Blobbing looked like fun."

"I think so."

"You missed a lot…being with me."

Sharon squeezed her hand. "I gained a lot more."

"Thanks."

"Thank you."

Vicky turned to Sharon. "Jesus said come to the water. I think
I'll be going to the water soon."

Sharon tried to respond, but couldn't. A surge of compassion
welled up within her, clutching at her chest. Tears streamed
down her face. Never before had she been involved so directly
with someone on the verge of leaving this life.

Camp Barnabas called me at work the morning of July 17. Vicky
bumped her knee on the dinner table, and could not walk. A blood test
showed that Vicky needed both red blood and platelets. I talked with
the doctors at children's hospital, and then called the staff at camp. It
was best for Vicky to finish camp by staying one more day. Vicky had
talked at length with Vanessa and I about camp. Vanessa and I were at
peace knowing that staying one more day was God's will.

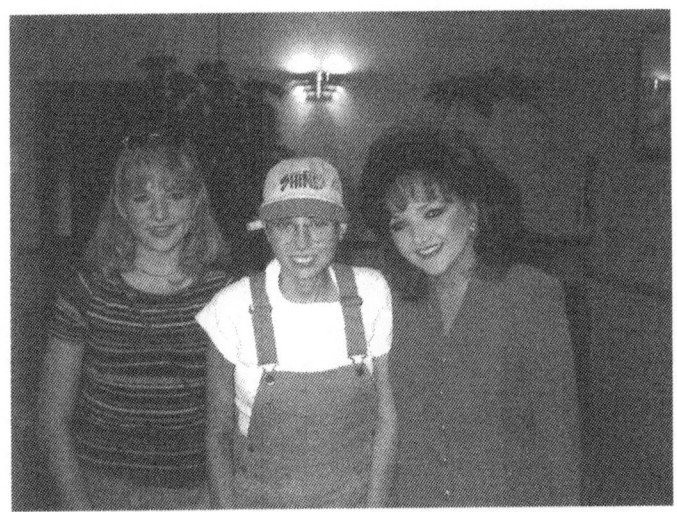

Vicky meets with Karen Wheaton (right) and her daughter Lauren

THE DESIRES OF HER HEART

Vicky was in bed at the infirmary when Vanessa and I arrived at camp Barnabas the afternoon of July 18. Sharon Reier was Vicky's personal counselor. Her sister, Jenn Reier, was the activity coordinator for the camp. Sharon put Vicky in her wheel chair, and wheeled her to the assembly area for award presentations. All of the families joined in with their kids for the presentations. Windle received an award for learning how to swim. All of the kids at camp received awards for their courage, endurance, and faith. Everyone was treated to a special song. The kids performed skits the night before camp closed. One of these performances was presented for the families. Jenn, Sharon, and Vicky sang the song: "Friends." Everyone was moved to tears as Vicky struggled to endure the heat while breathing deep enough to get the words out. Vicky was then awarded the Hosea 6 award for enduring to the end. The families then went to each cabin where more special awards were presented to all of the campers. Addresses and phone numbers were exchanged before families headed home for the weekend.

Saturday was spent unpacking and rehearsing the events of camp. Windle was very excited, but Vicky was very tired. Vicky was scheduled for transfusions Monday, but she was wishing it were now. Vicky's appetite was gone along with her energy. She spent most of the day in bed.

The family went to church Sunday morning. Vicky was so tired that she lay on the pew. She was complaining of her side hurting again. When she sat up to go home, Vicky nearly passed out. It was obvious that her red blood count was too low. She was pale and lifeless. Vanessa and I rushed Vicky to the emergency room at Arkansas

Children's hospital. An ultra sound of Vicky's gall bladder showed it to be normal, but still full of stones. The illius on the colon was still visible. She was transfused with two units of red blood, and placed in a room on the bone marrow transplant unit since all other rooms were full. A x-ray of the right knee was normal. I took Windle and Stacy back home while Vanessa stayed with Vicky.

Vicky needed three more units of red blood and two units of platelets Monday morning. Friends from church came to visit with Vicky. Her side was hurting so much that she was not able to enjoy the visit. Another ultrasound was done to check the gall bladder in preparation to remove it. Vicky was placed on a clear liquid diet in preparation for surgery.

Vicky was returned to a normal low-fat diet Tuesday in order to gain strength prior to surgery to remove the gall bladder. I took off from work to consult with the surgery team. The surgeon told Vicky that the decision to remove the gall bladder was up to her. Tears welled in her eyes, and then she demanded that it be removed now! Surgery was scheduled for Thursday afternoon.

Vicky was moved Wednesday to the surgery ward, called 3 Orange. The surgery team checked Vicky one more time. They were not convinced that Vicky's pain was coming from the gall bladder. The surgery was put on hold, and the pain team was called to evaluate Vicky's pain. Vicky's weight was down to 97 pounds, and she was not eating. The doctor told Vicky that he would put the feed tube back in if she did not start to eat.

The pain team came in Thursday morning to work with Vicky. The team selected oxycodone to see if Vicky's pain was in the muscles. There were specific medications to control pain in the nerves, in the muscles, and in the internal organs. The pain team started with the muscles since this appeared to be the location of Vicky's pain. The mediation made Vicky's pains go away. The surgery to remove Vicky's gall bladder was canceled. The pain team wanted to keep Vicky in the hospital over the weekend for physical therapy and fine tune adjustment of the pain medication. The feed tube was put in at Vicky's request.

Vicky's white blood count started falling Friday. Her platelet level was also low, and she received two units of platelets. The physical therapist performed relaxation massage to Vicky's stomach muscles. This helped to reduce her pain, and lower the dosage of oxycodone needed to control pain. I brought Windle and Stacy to Little Rock for the weekend, and checked into a motel. Vanessa stayed the night in the motel with the family. Vicky called three times during the night to tell Mom and I that she was feeling much better.

Vicky's white blood count was still low on Saturday. I asked doctor Saylors about restarting the GCSF injections. Doctor Saylors stated that patients who were treated for Ewing's sarcoma keep low blood levels for a long time. Their platelet level will stay below 15 for up to eighteen months, and the white count will stay around 1 to 1.5. The physical therapist helped Vicky walk and exercise her arms. When the therapist massaged Vicky's stomach there were knots in the muscles. The therapy made the knots go away. I took Windle and Stacy back home at night.

After church, I left Windle and Stacy with a family, and I went to Little Rock. Vicky said that she was having a great day. Vanessa sat on one side of Vicky and I on the other. Vanessa and I took turns helping Vicky with all kids of crafts that provided physical therapy to her arms. I headed back home to pick up Windle and Stacy. Vanessa called me just as I got home to ask about a bump on Vicky's head. I was sitting on the side the bump was described to be on. Vicky did not remember hitting her head. Vanessa showed the bump to the nurse.

Vicky's head was x-rayed early Monday morning. The x-ray looked normal. A long acting version of Vicky's new pain medication was started. Vicky could go home in the morning as soon as the blood level for the pain medication was in a normal range. I received a call from the water department. The meter was read in the morning, and it showed a four-time increase in the normal water usage. I left work to find the problem. I isolated the leak between the meter and the house. I dug up the water line at the meter and under the house, but no leak was found. I called a friend at church, and the two of us replaced the water line between the house and the meter in the rain. It was late at night before I was finished.

Vicky's bump on her head was bigger Tuesday morning. A CT scan of the skull was performed. The skull was moth-eaten, and a tumor was growing into the brain. Radiation to the site was scheduled to start Thursday. Doctor Becton said that the skull is a major source of bone marrow. Therefore only enough radiation to stop tumor growth would be administered. A phase-one chemotherapy drug would be tried in two weeks if Vicky's white count would increase. There was concern that the cancer was in the bone marrow. Vicky was given a zero percent chance of survival, and only a 50 percent chance of response to the chemotherapy. The chemotherapy would drop Vicky's white count to zero for such a long time that she was given a 90 percent chance of dying because of an infection. Doctor Becton would talk to the family at length on Thursday. During the evening Vicky's neck started getting sore. Later that night her right arm went numb along with her lower lip and chin. Vicky started biting her lower lip to try to restore some feeling. The lip started bleeding and would not stop. The blood level was checked, and her platelets were at 5. Cold compresses were needed to stop the bleeding.

Vicky was transfused with two units of red blood and one unit of platelets early Wednesday morning. Vicky's white count was still going down. Vicky started experiencing severe chest pains. A chest x-ray was ordered. There was concern that Vicky's white count was falling because of pneumonia. Vicky's lower teeth hurt every time she chewed or drank anything cold. Sharon Reier called Vicky and said that she was flying in from Minnesota next Thursday to spend 5 days in the hospital with Vicky. Sharon Reier was Vicky's personal counselor at Camp Barnabas, and she was scheduled to be back at camp Monday, August 4. But, all counseling positions filled up, and Sharon was told not to come. When Sharon heard of Vicky's diagnosis, she felt God leading her to go to Vicky. Sharon changed her flight schedule to spend five days at the hospital with Vicky. Vicky started looking forward to Sharon's visit.

Vicky woke Thursday morning with a cough. Vicky and I rode Angel 3 to CARTI for radiation treatments. Vicky would receive 400 Rads for 5 days to the skull. The energy level was low enough that brain damage would not occur. Vicky asked to visit with Jennifer while at CARTI. Jennifer and Vicky visited for a while and then went to the toy closet. Vicky returned with a stuffed bear named "Pedington." Sharon Reier called Vicky and said that the plane ticket was in hand. Some of Vicky's friends from camp Barnabas called and said that they were coming to visit with Vicky on Sunday.

Brother Dade and Sister Sheila joined Vanessa and I to talk with Doctor Becton and Gregg Adams. There appeared to be two masses growing out of the thickening of the lung lining into the left lung. Other tumor spots were expected to crop up nearly every day. The radiation to the skull may not kill the tumor. The energy level was low enough to allow for total absorption in the bone. Chemotherapy was no longer an option. Full strength chemotherapy would kill Vicky. Vicky was given two to three weeks to live. The oxygen level would slowly drop and carbon dioxide levels will slowly increase. This meant that Vicky's energy level would constantly drop, and she would sleep more and more. Terry was in the room when Doctor Becton rehearsed all the information with Vicky. Terry could not hold back his emotions. Vicky did not know what to think about everything. She was sure she wanted to go home as soon as she could, but she did not want to die at home. She wanted to be in the hospital when she died. Vanessa was very upset. Vanessa, Terry, and I went home to let everyone sort things out.

Gregg Adams talked at length with Vicky on August 1st. Windle and Stacy were left with friends, and Vanessa and I went back to Little Rock. Vicky asked Gregg if she could go to 6 Flags or Disney World. Gregg told Vanessa and I that another dream could not be funded. Vicky and I rode Angel 3 to CARTI for the second radiation treatment. Vicky was very tired, and slept most of the afternoon. Vanessa was very stressed, and had a bad headache. The nursing staff found a quiet room for Vanessa to lay in.

The lab report showed a gram-positive bacterial infection growing in Vicky's blood Saturday morning. Two different antibiotics were started. Vicky needed another unit of platelets. Two families from church came to visit with Vicky. Kara Travis' mom and brother visited with Vicky. Vicky noticed a lump the size of a pea just below her ribs. The area around the tail bone started swelling. Vicky's energy level was going away quickly as expected.

Vicky was laying in bed when five counselors from camp Barnabas came to the hospital Sunday morning. There were Kevin Golden, Mary Grace, Jenn Reier, and two other boys. The group started singing before getting to Vicky's room. Vicky was smiling from ear to ear when the group busted into the room. Bulletins were handed out to everyone in the room, and church started. Each counselor read their part while the other counselors helped them "preach." And, preach they did for over an hour. Vicky loved it. A basket of toys and gifts was then presented to lift up her spirits. Vicky responded in a very positive manner, and the hospital staff was amazed. The group then asked Vicky to join them as they sang "Friends." Jenn and Mary painted Vicky's fingernails purple while Kevin painted his purple also. Vicky loved the special attention given to her. Vicky was handed a can of spray string, and then doctor Becton was called to the room. Doctor Becton was covered in string, and Vicky was having a blast helping. Vicky was prayed for before the group headed back to camp Barnabas. The counselors stayed three hours. Kara's mom visited in the afternoon. Vicky told her all about the events of the day, and encouraged her to send Kara to camp Barnabas. One unit of platelets was transfused. The follow up blood test showed that the white count had spiked up. Vicky said it was because of the power of prayer.

Vicky needed two more units of red blood Monday morning. I went to work, and Vicky rode Angel 3 to CARTI with her nurse. Rhonda heard about the events from Sunday, and checked on Vicky. Rhonda noticed that Vicky was much better.

On Tuesday, August 5, Vicky rode Angel 3 to CARTI with her nurse. When she got back to the hospital she was moved to the cancer ward with Rhonda as her nurse. Rhonda checked the knot on Vicky's head, and it was gone. The knot below the ribs stopped growing. The swelling around the tailbone went down. Vicky was much more alert, and enjoyed having Rhonda as her nurse. Vicky needed one unit of platelets. The man who bought Vicky's prom dress showed up in Vicky's room just as I got in from work. He said that God sent him, and then he prayed that Vicky would have the desires of her heart. Vicky gave him a signed copy of her book, and he left. Vanessa and I stepped into the hall to talk with him, but he was gone. His words echoed in everyone's mind: "Grant her the desires of her heart." Without a doubt this man was a messenger sent by God—an angel.

Vicky had an appointment with doctor Nicholas Wednesday morning. He reminded Vicky to be very careful with her arm, and always wear her cast. Vicky then went to CARTI for her last radiation treatment. Later that night Vicky's friend, Kara Travis, died. Vicky was peaceful in knowing that Kara was interceding for her before God. Vicky knew that the two would see each other again in heaven. Vicky asked to be left alone while her and her nurse, Sandy, talked about death and dying.

On Thursday, Sharon arrived to stay with Vicky. Vicky said it would be a long slumber party. Vanessa, Stacy, Windle, and I moved into a motel so that Sharon could move in with Vicky. There was something about Sharon that told me that this was right. Vanessa and I met Sharon for only 30 minutes at camp Barnabas. Other than a few minutes on the phone we barely knew Sharon. Yet we felt confident giving the hospital permission for her to stay in Vicky's room for the next few days. Sharon's suitcase was filled with craft materials to last the week. Vicky and Sharon did crafts, held devotions, and had fellowship with each other. Sharon watched as Vicky received one unit of platelets.

Vicky found out that Sharon's birthday was on Monday. Vicky requested, and obtained, a four-hour pass on Friday. Vicky took Sharon to Chuck E Cheese for a birthday party. Vicky made Mom and I promise to adopt Sharon and her family as our own. Vicky and Sharon were serious about adopting each other's family. Little did we know how real this adoption would be to everyone. Vicky then presented Sharon the Arkansas Children's Hospital "Ray of Hope" award. Vicky was excited to now have a big sister. Sharon and Vicky returned to the task of crafts, devotions, and fellowship. Vicky made plans to visit Sharon, her sisters Jenn and Laura, and her mom and dad in Minneapolis during an October school break. Sharon's mom, Carole, told Vicky that she could come at anytime. Vicky transfused three units of red blood during the night while the two girls stayed up for a slumber party. Sharon was starting to get use to the sounds of IV poles beeping during the night.

"Sometimes in our lives we are lucky enough to be touched by true angels.

Thank you, Sharon, for being that guardian angel, providing hope and inspiration, and going that extra distance to put everything in the proper perspective.

It is with grateful appreciation for your friendship and love that I present this

RAY OF HOPE AWARD

On this eighth day of August 1997.
Thank you for giving so much to me."

Vicky Bowen

Vicky's platelets were low again Saturday morning and she received one unit of platelets. Paula and Jennifer came to visit. Vicky was excited telling them about having a big sister. I took Sharon to dinner for her birthday. I asked Sharon why she felt God calling her to be with Vicky. Sharon shared all of the events in her life, and I shared all of the events in Vicky's life. I was very pleased to have Sharon as an adopted daughter.

Vicky's platelet level was 10 on Sunday morning, but red spots were showing up on her legs. She transfused one unit of platelets. Sharon left to meet her sister Jenn half way between Little Rock and camp Barnabas. Brother Dade and Sister Sheila visited with Vicky. They were amazed at the healing done in Vicky's body. I took Windle and Stacy home. Sharon and Jenn called to check on Vicky. They asked Vicky what she and the rest of the family wanted or needed. Sharon and Jenn took the list and went shopping at Wal Mart.

A package arrived at the hospital Monday morning. In it was a huge Teddy Bear from the Reir family. Sharon arrived at the hospital, and rolled in two large wagons full of wrapped gifts. Vanessa received slippers and an 8-place dish set. Vicky received a Pooh hat, purse, and cloths. Vanessa called me, and had me bring Windle and Stacy to the hospital for their gifts. Vicky asked me to open my present first. I was able to take pictures of Windle and Stacy opening their gifts with a new camera. When Sharon went home Monday, August 11, Vicky was walking, eating, and working crafts all day long. Vicky was walking in the middle of God's fifteen-day miracle of healing.

Rick Washam, one of my coworkers called me, and said that he stood in for Vicky during a healing service Sunday. After 30 to 45 minutes he felt the release that Vicky was healed. When Rick heard of all the events that happed during the week, he was humbled by the awesome presence of God's power.

On Thursday, August 12, Vicky wanted to make plans to see Karen Wheaton again. I checked, and Karen was scheduled to be in Branson over the upcoming weekend. The last time Vicky was in Branson, she wanted to ride the amphibious Ducks, but there was not enough time. Vicky needed two units of red blood and one unit of platelets. Vicky's gall bladder acted up, and she became nauseated. Feeds were stopped for the night.

On Wednesday, August 13, Vicky decided that she was going to leave the hospital and go to Branson to ride the Ducks and see Karen. Then she was going to Minneapolis for a slumber party with her adopted sisters, and going shopping at the Mall of America. I had no idea how to afford such a trip.

When I returned to work many of my coworkers donated a day of their vacation. There was enough vacation for me to take the whole year off if I needed to. My coworkers had also taken up a collection. There was enough money to make the trip to Minnesota. I realized that God was working in many different parts of the country at the same time on behalf of the desires of Vicky's heart.

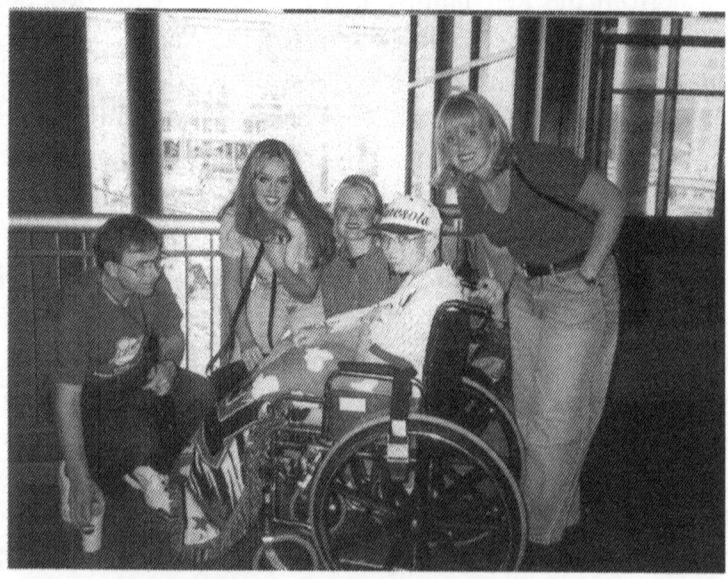

Vicky, Tom, and her three adopted sisters at the mall. Laura (left),
Sharon (center), and Jenn (right).

THE EAGLE'S FLIGHT HOME

Vicky's weight was up to 112.5 pounds, a gain of 15 pounds since admission. A knot above and to the left of the left breast showed up early in the morning. Vicky said it did not hurt, and she refused to show it to any of the nurses. Vicky wanted to start her trip on time. I knew that the cancer was in the lymph system. I wanted Vicky to live her last days her way and agreed not to tell the doctors. Vicky was discharged Thursday afternoon, and she spent the evening packing. During the night Vicky's nose started bleeding heavily because of the feed tube and a low platelet level. Vanessa packed while I helped stop the nosebleed. It took two hours for the bleeding to stop. I wanted to believe that Vicky would make the trip to Branson, but the bleeding started so quickly after being discharged from the hospital. What would I do if the bleeding started while in the motel? Who would I call? I refused to answer the questions and fell asleep at Vicky's side. Vanessa asked me to come to bed with her. I woke long enough to tell her that I was busy taking care of Vicky.

The trip to Branson started Friday morning with a stop at Arkansas Children's Hospital for two units of platelets. I wanted her to have more for the trip, but I new better than to ask. The doctors would ask why and the cancer in Vicky's arm would be noticed. I promised not to tell anyone.

As soon as Vicky got into the motel at Branson, she removed the feed tube. Vicky met Karen's daughter, Lauren in the lobby of the concert hall. Vicky got to hear David Ring preach after Karen sang. David Ring is a minister with cerebral palsy, and Vicky was impressed with his sermon and life story. Vicky bought one of David's hats that said: "Don't whine…Shine." Vicky resolved to give God the glory even if the cancer was not cured. Vicky asked to go out for dinner after the concert. Vicky asked me to promise to finish the book she started. She said that people needed to hear her story just like she heard David Ring's story. I promised to finish the book.

Saturday morning the family rode the amphibious Ducks. Windle drove the duck on the water. Stacy, Windle, and Vicky blew on their duck whistles the entire trip. Vicky ate ice cream and pizza for lunch. I was worried about her gal bladder acting up, but Vicky never did get sick. In the afternoon, the family moved into the motel Karen Wheaton was staying in. Vicky and Karen spoke on the phone at length, and Karen was amazed at the life in Vicky's voice. Karen, Lauren, and Vicky met in the lobby where Vicky received a beautiful teddy bear from Karen and an angel pin from Lauren. At the concert, Vicky heard Karen sing a song about running to the altar of God. Karen invited the family to a concert near Springfield the next weekend.

On Sunday, August 17, I drove the family to Kansas City. It took three hours to get out of Branson because of road construction. Vicky talked about David Ring's sermon, Karen's song about running to the altar, and Camp Barnabas. Vicky said that one day she would go running to God's throne, and say: "Here I am Lord, your faithful servant!" Vicky said that her and Jenn talked at camp Barnabas about being such a servant. Vicky ate fat-free lunchmeat and cheese sandwiches for dinner. Vicky's legs had red spots on them indicating the need for more platelets soon. I was really worried with the red spots showing. How much longer before a nose bleed would start? Where would I find a hospital for a platelet transfusion? Vicky's laughter and conversations eased my tension.

On Monday, the family arrived at Sharon's house in Minneapolis. Carole had dinner waiting for everyone. Sharon told her mom that Vicky liked fat free spaghetti without meat. Vicky was so excited telling everyone about her life story.

Vicky was determined to sleep in Sharon's bed. Sharon, Jenn, and Laura held a slumber party with their newly adopted sister. Vanessa, Stacy, Windle, and I were given the bottom floor of the Reier home. Vicky was glad to be adopted into such a loving family. I took the opportunity to hold Vanessa and talk about the days ahead. There was so much peace in the Reier home.

On Tuesday morning, Vicky woke up with a bruise on the side of her face where she slept on her hand. I knew that Vicky needed transfusions now. I called Minneapolis children's hospital and explained the situation. I was told that I could bring Vicky right away. Before going to the hospital, Vicky walked to the bathroom using her cane. Carole showed Vanessa and I the way to the hospital while Jenn stayed home with Stacy and Windle. Carole and Vanessa returned to the house, and Sharon and Jenn came to visit with Vicky. The hospital and clinic were very friendly. Doctor Susan Spencer was Vicky's oncologist while at Minneapolis Children's Hospital. Vicky needed both red blood and platelet transfusions. Vicky was exercising her right arm when her adopted sisters arrived. The arm had a knot near the shoulder. I thought that the cancer was growing. I showed Sharon the bump on Vicky's side. X-rays showed that the arm was broken at the area eaten away by cancer. Vicky apparently broke her arm when she bore her weight on her cane in the morning, but she never complained of any pain. Vicky's arm was put in a cast, and she put on Sharon's button up shirt. Stickers were immediately applied to the sling, and Vicky was Sassy to the core. Vicky's doctor at Minneapolis children's hospital pulled Jenn and Sharon aside. They were told of the manner in which most cancer patients die.

Back at Sharon's house, Laura painted Vicky's fingernails, and spelled out her name on both hands: VICKY BOWEN. After a dinner of spaghetti, Vicky asked to conduct the family devotion. The subject was the greatest gift: salvation. The girls made arrangements to go shopping at the Mall of America Wednesday. Carole, Vanessa and I spent the evening talking about Vicky's story and how Sharon, Jenn , and Laura got involved.

On Wednesday morning, Vicky took a bath, dressed, and rode to the mall in Sharon's car. Sharon had a license plate on the font her car naming it "Sassy." Sassy was riding in Sassy with Sharon and Jenn, and couldn't have been any happier. Carole rode with Laura, and Vanessa and I followed with Stacy and Windle. Vicky could not believe how huge the Mall of America was. She was ready to shop until her adopted sisters dropped. Vicky rode in the wheel chair while her adopted sisters took turns pushing.

The new, larger family spent nearly six hours at the mall. Vicky bought a shirt like Sharon's, a jacket, and a bath set. There was so much life in the mall. Death was the farthest thing from anyone's mind. Vicky reminded everyone that she had to get a gift for Sharon's boyfriend, Jeff. All but Carole and Laura arrived back at the house at 5:30 p.m. Vicky asked to lie on Sharon's bed again.

Vicky asked Mom to exercise her left foot, and I noticed that Vicky's knee was not up straight. Vicky said that she could not move her knee. Vicky then asked for someone to exercise her left hand, because she could not move it. Vanessa checked Vicky's right foot, and she could feel in that foot. But, Vicky could not feel anything on her left side. Then Vicky's speech started to slur. Vicky asked me if she was paralyzed, and I said yes. Vicky said OK, and asked me to rock her. My little girl was in my arms dying. Now what can I do? As I was rocking her, she gave me a big butterfly kiss. All I could think to do was call Doctor Stine at Arkansas Children's Hospital for instructions. Doctor Stine said to call 911, and remind them of the do not resuscitate order. While Vicky was waiting for the ambulance she asked to talk with Sister Sheila. Normally Sister Sheila was not home at this time of the day. Sister Sheila answered on the second ring. I told her that Vicky was dying and wanted to talk. Vicky listened on the phone as Sister Sheila talked and prayed with Vicky.

The paramedics started to load Vicky on the ambulance when she wanted to say good-bye to Jenn. I rode with Vicky while Vanessa and Sharon followed. Jenn kept Stacy and Windle. The ambulance ride seemed like minutes for me. Vicky was asking to move from her back to her side and back again. I was able to do something for Vicky. I knew how to roll her from side to side without hurting her fragile skin. For Vanessa and Sharon, the ride was an eternity. Vicky was quickly placed in a room, and vital signs were checked. The nurse could not find any pulse, no blood pressure, and no oxygen in the blood stream. Vicky's speech cleared up, and she asked to say good bye to Mom and her big sister, Sharon. I stood at the back of the room and watched. I didn't know what else to do. Vicky held onto Sharon's hand, and after 10 minutes Vicky took her last breath and closed her eyes. The desires of Vicky's heart were filled. It was the end of the fifteenth day from when the angel came to Vicky's room. I did not fully understand the significance of the fifteen days until I finished Vicky's book.

Sharon's dad, Ron, arrived with Laura at the hospital moments after Vicky died. Laura spent time in Vicky's room saying good bye to her adopted sister. I was asked if I wanted to go in with her. I couldn't go, and said that I had already said goodbye. I failed to realize that Laura needed me to be in the room with her.

Ron knew just who to call and what to do to get Vicky back home for the funeral. Sharon had asked Vanessa to bring Vicky's prom dress for a special occasion later in the week. Sharon took the dress to the funeral home. Vicky was dressed in her prom dress and blond wig. Windle drew a picture of Vicky in a wheel chair while everyone was gone. He said that he wanted to remember his sister having fun.

The new family ate breakfast together Thursday morning. Ron had special gifts for Windle and Stacy, and then let them sit in his patrol car. Sharon wanted to be at the funeral to take care of Vanessa and I, and say good bye to Vicky. Jenn wanted to be at the funeral to take care of Windle and Stacy, and also say good bye to Vicky. Laura wanted to

come, but she had obligations as the reigning Miss Teen Minnesota.
Ron made arrangements for Sharon and Jenn to fly to Arkansas.

Vanessa, Windle, Stacy, and I arrived home Friday afternoon. I took
the wheel chair off the back of the car and locked it in the trunk. I did
not want to see it in the mirror as I drove home.

Terry came home from college. Sharon and Jenn flew in Friday night.
Sharon, Jenn, and Laura really were adopted daughters who cared about
their sister. Visitation was held Friday night at the funeral home. Vicky
looked so beautiful and peaceful. There were so many visitors from my
work, Vicky's school, Terry's work, and the community. Vicky's angel
collection was set all around. Everyone noticed one special angel that
Terry bought the year before. The angel played "Amazing Grace."
Sharon and Jenn made sure their adopted family was made comfortable
before they went to bed.

The family ate lunch Saturday at Vicky's church. The ladies of the
church provided the meal. One of the camp Barnabas counselors, and
his roommates, met the family at the church. The funeral was at
Hartman cemetery at 2:00 p.m. Sharon and Jenn sang "Friends." I gave
an overview of Vicky's last journal. Dade Kindrix read from Matthew
18:10 about angels watching over children. He stated that Vicky's angel
would have to find someone new to watch over now because she was in
the presence of Jesus. I held tight to Vanessa while she held Stacy and
Windle. Sharon and Jenn stayed by Terry.

Sharon and Jenn headed for home Saturday night, and the rest of the
Bowen family went to Springfield to visit with Karen Wheaton. Karen
sang Sunday night, and ministered to the family. Karen especially spent
a season of prayer with Vanessa. At the end of the concert, Karen told
the story of Vicky and sang her favorite song: "Promise." Karen stated
that Jesus kept his promises to Vicky. Two people were saved, and over
20 families asked for healing in their homes. Vicky's servant attitude
was still ministering to people.

I drove the family home Monday, and started the process of putting the pieces back together. Wednesday was the hardest day when Vanessa and I went through Vicky's belongings. On Thursday, August 28, Vanessa and I took the rented medical equipment back to Little Rock. Vanessa and I shared are thoughts all the way to Little Rock. While there, Vanessa and I visited Children's hospital and the Open Arms apartment. Everyone was so glad to know that Vicky and God controlled all the events in her life. Several had not heard that Vicky died.

As you can see, miracles do happen today. By God's grace, the rest of the family will join Vicky in heaven one day. And it was Vicky's wish that all of her friends would join her in heaven one day also. Vicky wanted her peers to hear her story.

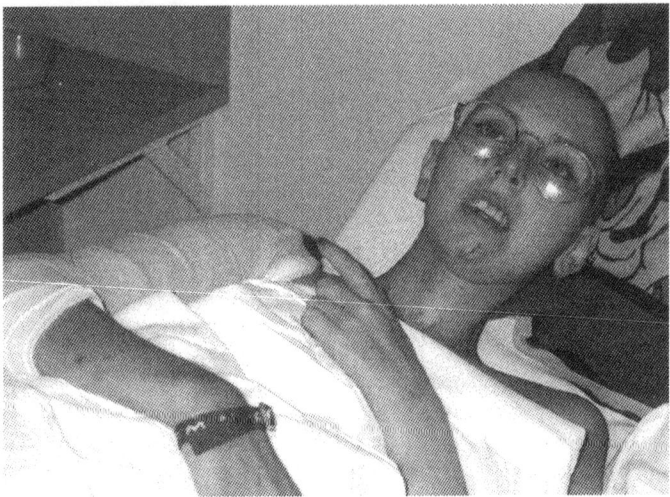

The cast was put on Vicky's arm at Minneapolis Children's

SUBMITTED WRITINGS

I would love to do away with some major painful, embarrassing, frustrating, even difficult events in my life. I would like to erase the pain and suffering Vicky experienced. I would like to remove the hurt her family bore. I would like to eradicate the tears and sorrow of that time when Vicky was so sick, and when she died. Given the opportunity, would I do away with these times? In the most critical times, God shows us his faithfulness in concrete ways.

Those two painful years when Vicky was dying—surely I would like to do away with those! But wait: there is the way God wrapped his arms around us all and comforted us; the love extended by friends and the body of Christ; the deep ways God revealed himself, and the lessons he taught us. I reflect on my changing view of heaven, how precious, real, wonderful it is to me because of Vicky and a little girl named Elizabeth there. I visualize Vicky and Elizabeth laughing, singing, and delighting in their home in heaven now.

Even if I could, would I dare purge the events that seem horrible, unfair, and painful to others and to me? And if I could, despite my limited view, I would not erase the deeper lessons that pain, suffering, frustration, sorrow, and—yes—even death bring. Can I not trust God with those events that still make no sense to me?

I am willing to put all the moments of my life, good and bad, understandable and incomprehensible, into the hands of God, who says his ways are perfect.

There are Angels everywhere and Vicky and Elizabeth were two angels that I know! But, no one can see, except those who were meant to be.

Sheila Kindrix
October 5, 1997

A Servant's Heart

When I passed through the gates of Camp Barnabas on June 3rd, 1996, little did I know that my life and my family's lives would never be the same. I have never been molded and stretched in so many ways by God as I have been at camp. I came home from camp last summer sharing nothing but inspirational, life changing stories which I had experienced first hand. My family and I shared laughter and tears when I told story after story how special children had impacted my life. God knew these stories were a foreshadow of a privileged experience my family would soon be called by God to serve in.

I remember calling Sharon a few days before she came down to camp to tell her about Vicky, her camper, and soon to be very special friend. I watched Sharon and Vicky both experience Camp Barnabas for their first time. Their friendship grew closer day by day. Sharon developed a passion for Vicky. I didn't mind sharing my older sister. I also didn't mind gaining a younger sister. Sharon is a role model in my life, and I knew she would be a perfect example to Vicky. God knew who he was picking when he placed Sharon with Vicky. I wish I would of gotten the chance to tell Vicky that she couldn't of asked for a better older sister, but there is no doubt in my mind that Vicky figured that out on her own. Sharon and Vicky shared a bond nobody will ever be able to replicate.

When I received the news Vicky and her family were coming to Minnesota, I was thrilled. I thought to myself, "Wow, Camp Barnabas at my house!" My family served Vicky and her family just like each one of the counselors did this summer at camp by putting others before themselves. They wanted to give to Vicky and her family with the same heart Vicky had—a servant's heart.

I had shared with my family something Vicky had shared with me. I can still picture us sitting in the infirmary the last evening of camp. I told Vicky that I was going to do an evening talk about Heaven. During our conversation I had asked Vicky what was the first thing she was going to say to Jesus. She thought about it and without hesitation she responded, "Here I am as your servant Lord." I was completely blown away. Here I stood next to Vicky, 21 years old, cancer free, and I had to ask myself if that would be the first thing I would say to Jesus. It proved to me that Vicky's faith in God was so strong. Looking at her lying in the infirmary bed, weak, dying at age 17, I was speechless. It taught me that my faith is like a child. In everything I do, I need to do it the way Jesus would do. Jesus was a servant. He washed his own disciples' feet. Vicky was an imitator of God.

I will always cherish the privilege of sharing the last month of Vicky's life with her. Because of the impact Vicky made on my life I am finishing school to become a child life specialist. And because of that, there is no doubt in my mind that I will come across many more "Vickys" in my lifetime. No one will ever be able to take the place she has stolen in my heart. My life will never be the same since I've been touched by an angel. She has touched so may people; Sharing her testimony still impacts people's lives. Vicky was a one of a kind. She was a fighter, an inspiration, and a servant. Vicky is in a place right where she's always dreamed of being, surrounded by angels. She is healthy, walking, laughing, singing, and praising God. I can visualize her right now, kneeling before the throne of God, living what her heart told—a servant to God.

For where your treasure is, there your heart will be also. **Matthew 6:21**

Jennifer Reier
September 16, 1997

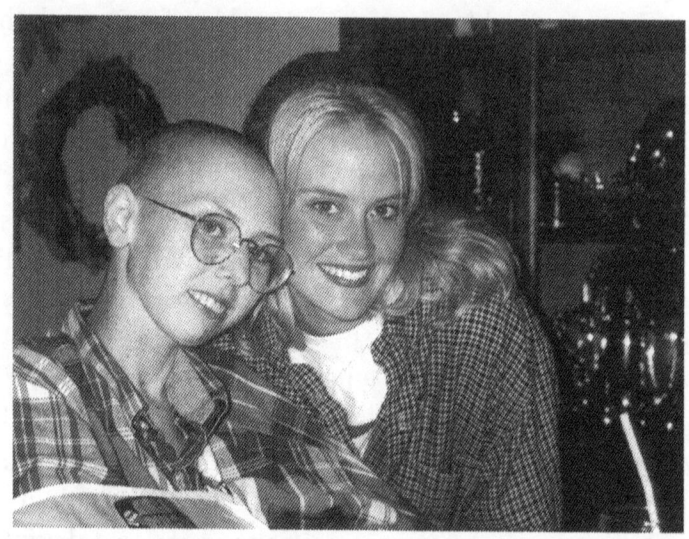

Vicky and her adopted sister Sharon. Vicky is wearing Sharon's shirt.

AND GOD SAID NO

I asked God to take away my pride. And God said "No."
He said it was not for him to take away, but for me to give up.

I asked God to make Vicky whole. And God said "No."
He said her spirit was whole, her body was only temporary.

I asked God to grant me patience. And God said "No."
He said patience is a by-product of tribulations. It isn't granted, it is earned.

I asked God to give me happiness. And God said "No."
He said he gives me blessings, happiness is up to me.

I asked God to spare me pain. And God said "No."
He said suffering draws you apart from worldly cares, and brings you closer to me.

I asked God to make my spirit grow. And God said "No."
He said I must grow on my own. But, he will prune me to make me fruitful.

I asked for all things that I might enjoy life. And God said "No."
He said I will give you life, that you may enjoy all things.

I ask God to help me love others, as much as he loves me.
And God said, "Ah, finally you have the idea."

Billy Lewis
October 1, 1997

ANGELS

There are **ANGELS** everywhere,
But, no one can see,
Except those who were meant to be.

You say unto me, "Look at the **ANGELS!**"
Then I began to wonder if you were in danger.

Only minutes passed by and turned into months,
Now only the good Lord has your touch.

Be with me always and show me you're near,
So I may never fear,
Of the **ANGELS**.

To my very special friend Vicky Bowen

Amanda Morrow
August 22, 1997

Forever Friends

Meeting Victoria on July 10, at Camp Barnabas was a day that God had obviously planned, and a day that would change my life forever! Vicky and I were set up to work one on one with each other, and that was the start to a beautiful, precious friendship. We spent many hours and days together, talking, laughing, praying, and most of all playing. Vicky had captured a special place in my heart. A place that no one before has ever found.

At camp, Vicky ministered to me by being a fighter and by completely trusting in God for His will to be done in her life. She wanted to be used by God, and she was his servant. What an awesome young woman of God!! She told me of her stories of seeing angels and Jesus, and how close to heaven she had been. We learned so much of each other over those days. I think my most precious memory of camp was singing "Friends" with her and Jenn. "Friends are friends forever…" That song describes us to a T!!

The last day of camp was sad, saying good-bye to my new precious friend, not knowing when and if I'd ever see her again. God had a plan for me two weeks later, and I didn't even know it!!

On August 7th, I flew into Little Rock and spent 4 1/2 days with Vicky. They were the greatest! It was over those four days that our friendship turned from the greatest of friends to the best of friends. We became sisters. I adopted Vicky and she adopted me. We spent hours doing crafts, reading, and talking (about everything). I got to sleep right next to her and we had a slumber party. It was so special to have Vicky take me out for a special birthday lunch and then give me the "Ray of Hope Award." What an honor!! It was hard to say good-by to Vicky on the 11th; not knowing what God had in store for her life. Once again, He was going to bless my life with her (and her awesome family) by letting them come to Minnesota.

She wanted to come up and see where I lived. I told her to come whenever but, for sure next summer for what I hoped to be my wedding.

Well, Vicky wanted to come now, and I'll never forget what she said to me on the phone the night before she arrived in Minneapolis. "I promised you I'd come Sharon, and I could never break my promise to you." And she had called me her sister. What an honor to have her and her family come all the way to see me and my family. I waited anxiously for their car to come around the corner, and at 7:15 p.m. Monday, August 18th; Victoria and her family were finally here!! The next two days would become the most precious days ever. We spent Monday night catching up, and laying in my room talking. Although she was low on blood, her spirit was still very strong. Tuesday, she spent the day in the hospital. Before she left, she had to have a hug from her "big sister." Jenn and I tried to entertain her and keep her spirits up. That night she spent with my family and Jeff, and we got to know and love her more and more. She read devotions to us and shared about the "treasure" we have in God. What an awesome way to spend her last night with her.

The next morning she continued to be bound and determined to shop. I was so honored to spend her final minutes with her. The fact that she wanted me to go to the hospital and hold her hand meant the world to me. I remember telling her how much I loved her, how she was my sister, and my most special friend in the world. And while she was going home—taking her final breaths, I told her to go home to Jesus and she was gone.

It has been an honor and privilege to call Victoria not only my friend but also my sister. God has blessed me with so many precious memories that I will always hold very near and dear to my heart.

I love you Victoria and I will always remember my "Vicky smile." And "a life time is not to long, to live as friends." Thank you for blessing my life.

Sharon Reier
August 22, 1997

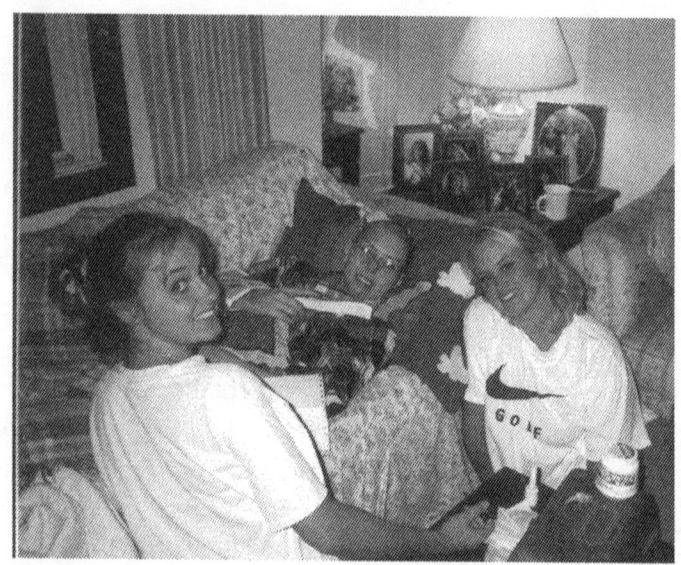

Laura (left) and Sharon (right) visiting with their adopted sister,

Lord:

When she was born,
I wondered if there had been a mistake!
How could something so precious belong to me?

And as she grew
Lord, so did I!
And everyone around us could see.

Now today
I have more riches than I ever dreamed I would have
Knowing one of your angels
for a while called me dad.

In my life
I have seen the miracle of love.

For, you sent an angel to me.
And I hope that you are pleased
with the care that I've shown.

Lord:

Please hold out your hands and shine your light
For I am giving back to you
what was never really mine to own.

Her life has been my finest hour.
I see her walking tall and on her own.
Lord hold out your hands.

For, I am sending my little angel home.

Now I know
that the tasks on your behalf for me are not quite through

But, dear Lord,
when you prepare her place...
please make room for two.

I believe that Vicky has changed my heart and soul.

I wrote this on the way back from seeing her on August 22, 1997.

Thank you,

Debbie Cole

In Memory of Sassy

I know that you're hurting
From the loss of your loved one.
Just know the Lord has her
In His strong arms and hands.
But, she is no longer hurting, and
her soul is at peace—
But, she knows how you miss her
and she *understands*.

Think of the joy you had—in
her living
And let the cool waters flow—
gentle and free.

You know you will see her
In God's Beautify Heaven
And,—*what* a Re-Union of love
that will be.

From Ruby Kennedy (Betty Robertson's mother)

THE TWO CROWNS

As we sat on the sofa, I painted Vicky's nails perfectly with her favorite color purple. I remember looking at her hands. Hands that were the same age as mine, but yet were pruned and discolored with a yellow-purplish tint. Vicky and I were alike in so many ways. We both were seventeen, and were going through the same stages of life. We were both in the same grade in school, loved to do make-up and paint our nails, go shopping, and do all the other things that normal teenage girls love to do. But, from the inside out we were in totally different worlds.

Thoughts spun around my head that morning as I did my daily routine of getting myself ready for the day. I was capable of taking care of myself and needed no assistance. Vicky's dad was the one that got her ready. He bathed her, dressed her, and would help her get comfortably situated in her wheelchair. I recall curling my long hair that morning and daydreaming about how beautiful Vicky must have been when she had long hair like mine. Instead, the chemotherapy and radiation had taken away all her hair and she was completely bald.

Vicky's body lay frail and almost lifeless. Her skin was pale with purple-yellowish blotches, which were caused from being touched in the most gentle way. It was a struggle for Vicky to live each day as she fought to take each breath. My life was focused around sports, pageants, and always being active. I had been working on my golden summer tan and losing that five extra pounds for my swimming suit to fit perfectly. In Vicky's life this was not necessary; cancer stole away the pounds.

We both had high hopes and dreams for our futures. I wanted to be Miss America someday and then marry a rich doctor and start a family. Vicky had the great hopes of being a pediatrics nurse, specializing in oncology. But for now, her greatest dream was to have a healthy life.

I watched Vicky that very same day as she struggled for her last few breaths. As we arrived at the hospital just minutes after the ambulance, I knew it was over. And, it was. The sad look of death had been painted across her parents' and my sister's faces. I walked into Vicky's hospital room to say my very last good-bye. She lay there cold, lifeless, but yet so peaceful. I was reaching for her cold clammy hand when I saw her purple nail polish that I had painted on her nails, and was reminded of all those special times that our families had together with Vicky. I knew that Vicky was in a better place. A place where there is no pain, no struggling, and no more cancer. She was finally in heaven rejoicing with God. Vicky no longer needed her wheelchair or for anyone to take care of her.

The next day, I had an obligation to be in a parade for currently holding the title of Miss Minnesota Teen. I forced a smile upon my face as I waved and greeted the crowds on the street. As the sun started to set, my thoughts were upon Vicky. Tears began to ponder as I asked myself why

I am here living this life of glamour instead of Vicky? How come she had fought a life full of cancer instead of it being my life? Then I was reminded of our heavenly crown that we will each receive when we pass through those gates of heaven. Vicky's crown that she was now wearing was a hundred times bigger and more spectacular than mine and would be with her for the rest of eternity.

I look forward to the day when Vicky and I will meet again. We will no longer be faced with all those differences, but instead live together happily in eternity.

Submitted by Laura Beth Reier,
Miss Teen Minnesota
June 17, 1998

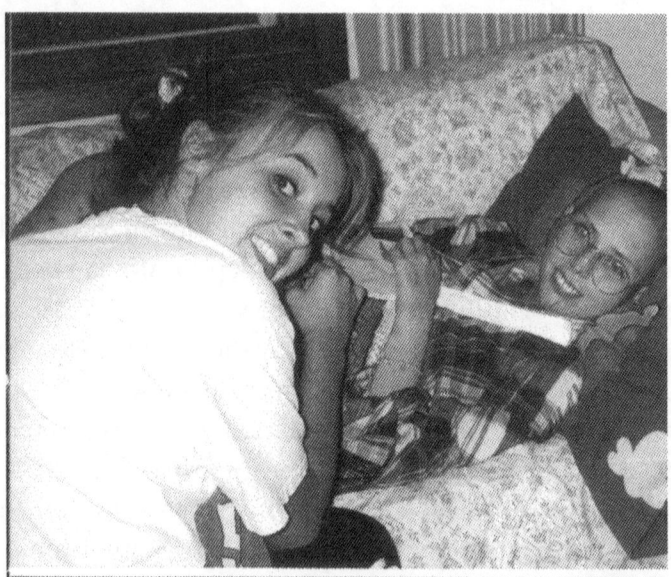

Vicky's adopted sister, Laura, painting finger nails.

ANGEL WATCHING OVER US

I know an angel who was once a great person and friend on this earth.
She was very Valuable in love.
No matter how much love she gave out, she still had plenty more
to share.
She was an Innocent girl, who never meant any harm to anyone,
and was always cheering someone up with her smile.
She always listened to you, whether you were griping about someone,
or telling her your painful stories.
She loved to talk—she was always telling some kind of story.
She was Caring and Kind-hearted.
She always put herself last, and God first,
and she was always thinking about the angels watching over us.
The worst part was that she was so Young.
She never had a chance to experience the "real world."
She had such a short time on this earth—she was only just starting,
but now she's up in Heaven, as healthy and happy as can be,
looking down on us, living an eternal life with our Father, and His
unlimited love.
Now it's her turn to be the ANGEL WATCHING OVER US.

To Vicky, with love
Ryan Youngblood
September 1997

Christ has redeemed me
from the curse of the law. Therefore,
I forbid any sickness or disease
to come upon this body.
Every disease germ and every virus
that touches this body dies instantly
in the name of Jesus.
Every organ and every tissue of this body
functions in the perfection
to which God created it to function,
and I forbid any malfunction in this body,
in the name of Jesus.
For greater is He that is in me
than he that is in the world.

Author unknown

Don't Worry, Everything's Going to Be Okay
By Collin McCarty

I know it hasn't been easy.
But you've done a pretty good job of hanging in there
and taking things day by day.

And I want you to remember…
Things are going to get better soon.

And because you are the special person you are,
I don't think it's going to take very long.

I want to give you every bit of encouragement
I possibly can. Believe in yourself
because you really are wonderful.

And don't forget that beyond the clouds
that sometimes get in your way,
the sun is shinning just for you…
and everything is going to be okay.

AFTERWORD

Grief counseling was provided through Arkansas Children's hospital. Until I was faced with this heavy grief I did not know what was acceptable or unacceptable reactions to this type of pain. I am so glad that Vanessa and I attended this training with our son, Windle. Stacy was considered too young for the training, and Terry was too busy with college to attend. When Stacy started kindergarten the teacher noticed possible learning disabilities. At the end of all of the evaluations it was identified that Stacy was in the midst of grief over the loss of her sister. The school used the counseling guide provided by Arkansas Children's hospital for both Windle and Stacy. The school noticed a significant change in Windle from before and after the counseling. Windle was still dealing with the grief. Vanessa and I were told that it takes from two to five years to recover from such a loss. The time element is correct. Everyone involved in the loss of a loved one needs to attend a grief class. I was relieved to find out that my feelings and emotions were normal. I also know to wait for Vanessa and my children to complete their process of grieving.

Vanessa and I knew that our visit to the Reier home was cut short by Vicky's death. I made arrangements to fly to Minneapolis after Christmas to finish the visit. Vanessa and I spent a week in Carole's home while Windle, Stacy, and Terry stayed home with friends. Carole knew exactly what was needed to help us heal. This godly woman gave priority to the words of comfort, the devotions, the music, and the moments alone. On New Years eve Jeff asked Sharon to marry him. We were all so excited. Vanessa and I made plans to return to Minneapolis for their wedding.

Our entire family made the trip to Sharon's wedding. Words alone could not describe our heart ache knowing that Vicky was not there, but yet she was there in everyone's hearts. Jenn's boyfriend, Abe, was at the wedding. Terry and Abe became best of friends. As we were ready to head home we were told that Carole was engaged to marry. We were so happy for Carole. The trip home was filled with conversations about the new larger family.

Windle attends camp Barnabas each year. His first return was in honor of Vicky. The "Victoria Bowen" award was presented to a camper struggling for life as much as Vicky did. Vanessa and I visited the cross overlooking the valley. Vicky's name was on the left side of the cross along with two other names of campers who died. Jenn told us that Abe visited her at camp and asked her to marry him. We were so excited for Jenn and Abe. We looked forward to another trip to Minnesota.

The entire family made another trip back to Minnesota for Jenn and Abe's wedding. Jeff assisted in the marriage ceremony now that he is a minister. Terry and I stayed at the reception until it closed. I will never forget the feelings I enjoyed when I danced with the bride. Jenn headed off to school to become a Child Life specialist to work with kids with cancer.

I made a trip to Shreveport for the Miss Teen USA pageant. Laura represented Minnesota at the pageant. I lost my voice screaming for the best girl on stage. Laura won the heart of her adopted dad. Visiting with Sharon and Carole at the pageant was awesome.

Our family visits with Karen Wheaton every year. Karen is a very special friend who takes time to pray, especially for Vanessa. Karen's music touches that special place in our hearts where Vicky's memory lives. Karen's music plays most nights when Vanessa and I go to sleep.

Vanessa and I wanted to help kids with cancer so much that we started a 501(c)(3) foundation. TAB Learning Systems, Inc is a foundation lifting the spirits of kids with cancer and other life threatening diseases and injuries. We focus on educating families, schools, and communities to the needs of kids with cancer. "Toys for Joys" is an annual fundraiser to put toys in the hands of caregivers at Arkansas Children's hospital. We want to raise enough funds each year to send kids to camp Barnabas and fill their dreams.

ABOUT THE AUTHOR

Thomas A. Bowen is a Level 3 Certified Control Systems Technician, and qualified instructor for the nuclear industry. Thomas earned his Bachelor of Arts in Education from Kingsway Christian College and Theological Seminary. He is presently working on an Electrical Engineering degree at Arkansas Tech University. Thomas holds active affiliation with the General Council of the Assemblies of God. Thomas is the founder and president of TAB Learning Systems, Inc., a foundation for listing the spirits of kids with cancer and other life threatening illnesses. Thomas is forty-eight years old and married 27 years to Vanessa. They make their home in Hartman, Arkansas along with three children.

References

Everyone's Guide to Cancer Therapy, by Malin Dollinger, Somerville House Books Limited, ISBN 0-8362-2427-2

This book covers all types of cancer and all types of treatments in understandable terms. Cost is $19.95.

Arkansas Children's Dreams Inc.
P.O. Box 7301
Little Rock, AR 72217

They are a state organization providing scholarships to kids with cancer.

Camp Barnabas
Rt. 2 Box 131
Purdy, MO 65734
(417) 476-2565
http://www.campbarnabas.com/

Friends Network
P.O. Box 4545
Santa Barbara, CA 93140
http://www.cancerfunletter.com

Friends network is a national activity letter for kids and families living with cancer. Annual cost is $10.00.

Karen Wheaton Ministires.
P. O. Box 1508
Hamilton, AL 35570
1.800.345.2736
http://www.KARENWHEATON.COM

Karing
Charlotte Hawkins
80601 Driver Rd.
Wamic, OR 97063

> Charlotte lost a child to cancer, and put this book together to help other families organize the volumes of information about treatment. Cost is $25.00

Ronald McDonald House
1009 Wolfe
Little Rock, AR 72202

> For a home away from home when you cannot stay in your child's room.

TAB Learning Systems, Inc.
Route 1, Box 304A
Harman, AR 72840
www.tablearning.org

> A 501(c)(3) Public Foundation lifting the spirits of kids with cancer.

TLC Foundation
6116 North Central Expressway, Suite 1400
Dallas TX 75206

> They are a Christian organization that can help families of seriously ill children.